The Art of Changing

GLEN PARK

The Art of Changing

Exploring the Alexander Technique
and its relationship to the
Human Energy Body

Illustrated by
DELIA HARDY

ASHGROVE PUBLISHING
London and Bath

With thankfulness to Don Burton
(1943 – 1996)

CONTENTS

AUTHOR'S NOTE AND ACKNOWLEDGMENTS

Ten years have passed since *The Art of Changing* was first published, and I am delighted that there is enough interest to warrant this new edition. When I first wrote the book I did wonder if it was appropriate to put all my developmental ideas about the Alexander Technique into a book which was essentially an introductory and explanatory book about the fundamental principles of the technique. Ten years further on my own life bears testimony to the need to understand and work with the emotional and energic patterns, which hold us in misuse. In the month the book was published I conceived twins and gave birth to two wonderful boys eight months later. The intensity of emotion I experienced as the parent of these two miracles of life was out of all proportion to anything I have experienced before. My feelings of joy, wonder and terror about the responsibility of being their parent were and still can be awesome. And the level of work involved in taking care of my twins was awesome too, especially as one of them had health problems which are only just beginning to recede.

I can say with pride that during those early years when I was carrying these two bouncing boys around, up and down stairs, in and out of cars, round and round the garden, my back stayed strong. I am only five foot two inches tall and I gave birth at forty-three years of age. Thank you F. M. Alexander for giving the world your discoveries. Through them, I have learnt the basic principles for taking care of my physical use. However, my anxiety levels soared especially when one of my children was ill, and my use deteriorated accordingly. So I realised how critically important it is for Alexander Teachers to work with emotional patterns of misuse, and not just physical ones, if we are seriously working with the whole self.

The teacher who showed me the importance of working with the whole self was Don Burton. His training courses offered students the freedom to really discover who they were, physically emotionally, mentally and spiritually, within the framework of the Alexander Technique. He supported my interest in psychic development and encouraged me to realise my potential. He himself was an inspired and brilliant teacher of the Alexander Technique, of anatomy and in the field of meditation. Without his influence and support this book could never have been written.

Delia Hardy has completely reworked the line drawings for this new edition and I am most grateful to her. Her skillful ability to clarify complex concepts visually, her commitment and enthusiasm were invaluable, in what proved to be a mammoth task. Jointly we dedicate this book to Don and to the growing seed he sowed in the Alexander world.

John Kennaby designed the cover, researched the photographs and computer-enhanced many of the images. He was there to help when the task became over-whelming, supporting me both as a versatile design consultant and a life partner! I wish to thank him from the bottom of my heart.

I am grateful to all the many teachers, and students* of the Alexander technique with whom I have worked and from whom I have learnt an immeasurable amount, and in particular to Felicity Columbi and Anne Turner for helpful comments and for our 'hands on' sessions together. My thanks also to teachers, therapists, colleagues and friends working in other disciplines for helping me to grow and change, to learn new skills and develop my own synthesis.

I wish to acknowledge Michael Symonds who was an extraordinarily gifted teacher of psychic skills who brought clarity and depth to my emerging psychic awareness. The latter part of this book draws largely upon his wisdom. Also, my appreciation goes to Ivy Northage and Wynn Kent who started me on the path of psychic development.

My thanks also go to my publishers, Robin Campbell and Brad Thompson for invest-ing time, energy and money to create this new edition.

Finally a big thank you to Chris and Joe for putting up with a Mum and Dad who were working nearly every weekend for two months. You were great. And thanks for just being there and demonstrating how much more fun life is, when we stop endgaining.

*I have used the word 'student' to cover teachers, trainee teachers and pupils throughout this book.

INTRODUCTION

Most people want to change something or other about themselves. It may be a physical problem. The first friend I ever made, when I was four years old, wanted, for as long as I can remember, to change her nose; eventually, in her thirties, she did have cosmetic plastic surgery. To her astonishment nobody noticed any difference when she emerged with her new nose. To all her friends she was just the same Linda. I think she felt it was worthwhile just to discover that, but it does beg the question of what we mean by 'change'.

When I was in my early teens I wanted to improve my posture and the way I moved. From a very early age I had extremely cowed and rounded shoulders, out of which my head and neck protruded in a very forwards direction. My back was hunched and very weak, so that from my early twenties I suffered from sciatica and low back pain. When I was at school it was my great ambition to receive a posture badge, and feel that I could look like the poised young women who sported them on their gymslips. I remember really trying to stand up straight and put my shoulders back. Alas, it worked! At the end of the year three names were called out for posture badges and one of them was mine. I raced up to the front of the school to receive it, my head stuck forward, my shoulders pulled round self-consciously to protect me from the attention. It just wasn't that easy to change. And I had tried pretty hard, which was part of my problem.

I had given up on my posture when I first began having Alexander lessons. I just wanted to be relieved from the constant bouts of back pain. So it was with great delight that I experienced the changes that took place. Friends would say to me 'You've changed. What's happened?'. When I asked them to describe the nature of the changes they would mention how much stronger I seemed, more confident, more open. The words they used suggested physical and psychological changes, changes which I also was noticing in myself. But this time I wasn't trying. My Alexander Teacher told me very little about the Alexander technique. But my body was listening and learning in a totally new way. It was getting an experience of a changed way of being, and because it liked it, it carried on being like that for as long as I would let it, before my old habitual interferences got in the way. I was learning how to move in a much more graceful and balanced way, something I had always longed to do. My posture altered dramatically, and it just seemed to be happening without a lot of effort.

Those times in our lives when we discover something very new and special and important to us, do not happen all that often. Discovering the Alexander Technique, the unfolding of its philosophy, the experiential nature of the learning and the attention to process rather than product was a very wonderful experience for me. Hitherto I had spent ten years working in the professional theatre, where the dominant theme was that the show must go on at all costs; and so to become involved in a technique that concerned itself with process was revelatory. More than that, the changes that took place in me as a result of a teacher putting her hands on my body were extraordinary. I cannot pass on that experience in a book but I hope I may encourage some readers to begin working with an Alexander Teacher. Ideally I would like this book to be used alongside the direct experience of Alexander work with a teacher.

The changes we want to make in ourselves may not be physical ones. We may want to change difficult personal character traits, bad habits that seem to rule our very being. Changing is an art, it cannot be rushed or forced. To try to do so will only lead to the sort of problems I experienced when I tried to change my posture. In Alexander's words, 'Change involves carrying out an activity against the habit of life'. The principles of the Alexander Technique can be applied to all aspects of our being. They are a method by which we can allow change to take place in ourselves, in an integrated way.

The first part of this book outlines the theoretical basis of the technique and at the same time allows the reader to experience some of these ideas practically. For the reader who has had several lessons in the technique I hope it will considerably enhance her* understanding and practice of it. It may be quite difficult for a person who has never worked with an Alexander Teacher to understand the nature of these observational exercises, and I would encourage anyone who is working with this book and who has never had lessons to see if they can find a teacher in their area, as the experience of working with a teacher will make a great deal of difference to the experience of reading this book.

When I began training to be an Alexander Teacher I was also extremely interested in other areas of the 'Growth' or the 'Human Potential' movement, in which the Alexander Technique plays its part. I trained in psychic development in England and

---

*In order to avoid being sexist I shall sometimes use the feminine pronoun and adjective (she, her, hers) to cover a general reference to a woman or a man, and at other times I shall use the masculine pronoun and adjective (he, him, his) to refer to both men and women.

California, and this has been of tremendous help to me in my work as a teacher. I see the Alexander Technique as a foundation upon which the rest of my work is based and from which it can grow and expand. In the second half of the book I have developed a synthesis between the Alexander Technique and my understanding of the human body as an energy system. I have also explored the area of human emotions in relation to the Alexander Technique. I see the second part of the book as an application and development of the principles of the Alexander Technique into areas which are of great interest and concern to many people.

How to use this book

1) For those readers who know nothing about Frederick Matthias Alexander (who developed the Alexander Technique), I recommend that you begin by reading the Appendix, which is a brief history of his life.

•2) Throughout the book I have suggested practical experiments, or observational exercises.† These are not 'exercises' in the sense that most people mean when they use the word. They are not like 'keep fit' exercises, or 'stretch' exercises. They are an opportunity to carefully explore aspects of yourself about which you may not be aware. They need to be carried out slowly and thoughtfully, with attention to the process of how you are doing them. The purpose of them primarily is to develop self-awareness.
   Read each exercise through carefully before beginning. The best way to work with the longer exercises would be to tape-record the instructions, leaving plenty of space between each instruction, so you have time to observe yourself without rush.

3) There is a CASSETTE TAPE which is available to accompany this book, on which I have talked through some of the exercises. On SIDE ONE of the tape there is a talk-through of things you can observe and think about when lying in the semi-supine position. (See Chapter Two, The Semi-Supine Habit)
   On SIDE TWO of the tape there is a talk-through (also for lying in the semi-supine position), which involves working with the Alexander Technique and the Chakras together.

†These sections are indented and marked by a dot (•) before and after the heading.

PART ONE

*F*UNDAMENTALS

Chapter One

The Use of the Self

It is what man does that brings the wrong thing about, first within himself and then in his activities in the outside world, and it is only by preventing this doing that he can ever begin to make any real change. (FMA,UCL)*

The last two books FM Alexander wrote were called *The Use of the Self*, and *The Universal Constant in Living*. What is universally constant in our living is the way we use ourselves. Our use is the way in which we do things in our daily lives, from the way in which we get out of bed in the morning, the way we stand up, sit down, or walk around, the way in which we do all the hundred and one activities of the day, to the way in which we lie down and go to sleep at night. We tend to go about the simple everyday acts of living in the same way, day in, day out. This concept of the 'use of the self' is central to Alexander's work, because he discovered a way in which we can continually improve our use in all that we do. And by learning to change our use we affect fundamentally every aspect of our experience.

Everything we do can be done in a good way that promotes healthy functioning or it can be done in a way that is harmful to our good functioning; that is, we can operate with good use, or we can misuse ourselves. Alexander discovered that we all share common habits of misuse, and the central purpose of Part One of this book is to explain what Alexander meant by misuse, what he meant by good use, and how we can learn to stop the misuses and allow a new improved use of the self to develop.

*Abbreviations used with quotes are as follows:

FMA Frederick Matthias Alexander
The four books written by Alexander:
MSI = *Man's Supreme Inheritance*
CCC = *Constructive Conscious Control of the Individual*
UOS = *The Use of the Self*
UCL = *The Universal Constant in Living*

Until Alexander made the discovery that our use affects our functioning there was no clear understanding of the importance of misuse as a reason for malfunctioning. The main reasons for malfunctioning were considered to be hereditary factors, on the one hand, and physical trauma on the other. For example, if you had a backache it was because you had inherited a weak back, or a weak constitution generally, or because something 'had happened' to your back which was causing it to malfunction, something like a car accident, or similar physical trauma. These are valid reasons for back pain, and there are excellent therapies for dealing with these problems. Nowadays we are aware that malfunctioning can be caused by many different factors in addition to heredity and physical trauma, such as emotional factors and dietary ones. What Alexander discovered was that one fundamental cause of back pain and of many other malfunctions is the way we use ourselves. In the course of his life Alexander worked with people suffering from a diversity of health problems, all of which improved as a result of learning the principles of his technique.

When a student comes to an Alexander Teacher with a problem such as a back pain, shoulder tension, a postural defect, a stress problem, or another of the many reasons that bring a student to this technique, the teacher's approach will not be to focus on the particular problem. The teacher may consider what the student is doing to cause the problem. Her concern will be with the use of the person, not with past traumas and problems, but with what is actually happening here and now. Specific problems are seen as manifestations of a more general dis-ease, the dis-ease of misuse. Although people often come to the Alexander Technique because they have a specific problem, Alexander Teachers do not claim to cure these problems. They offer to teach an improved use of the self, in the course of which the problem may clear up.

An Alexander Teacher can help you to understand how you are misusing yourself, and for a short time she can give you an experience of an improved use, but ultimately students must take responsibility for improving their own use, in their everyday lives. This opportunity to take responsibility for oneself is an important aspect of the Alexander Technique, and it is why we call ourselves teachers and not therapists, and why we work with students or pupils, not clients or patients. As soon as you understand that something you are doing may be causing your problems, then it is your choice whether you learn how to alter that situation or not. The teacher is there to help you make those changes if you wish to.

We develop habits of misuse because of the stresses and strains that we experience in our lives. In particular, Alexander emphasized that our modern society demands enormous and constant adaptations when compared to the lives of people living in a more natural environment. The rate at which change is occurring in our civilization is phenomenal, as new technology is introduced and older technology is discarded. One noticeable change for most Western people is that the mental aspects of life have become increasingly dominant, and the physical ones less essential, and so our lives have become comparatively sedentary and mentally oriented. Because of this we are more in touch with our minds and less in touch with our bodies (insofar as it is possible to separate the two). In Alexander's words:

'Mental' growth continued even after a deterioration had been recognized in the 'physical' self, and this deterioration caused, as it were, one limb of the tree to grow at such a pace that it over balanced the tree, bent it too much in one direction, seriously disturbing the roots responsible for its equilibrium and healthy growth. (FMA, CCC)

The nature of our complex civilized society is mirrored in our own nervous systems. There is a constant demand to adapt to a changing environment, and this creates stress, excitement and over-stimulation. There seems to be too little time for the nervous system to calm down and undo the stresses we have been dealing with, and so the stress responses take on a chronic pattern because they do not have time to release. The way we respond to our environment differs from individual to individual, and whereas one person may be hyperactive, another may be chronically depressed and lethargic, and another may suffer acute back pain or some other dis-ease. All these extremes show an inability to balance the demands on the nervous system, and can often be traced to habitual patterns of misuse.

The Alexander Technique teaches you how to release these chronic patterns of misuse, not only when you are at home, recovering from the trials of the day, nor simply during the period of an Alexander lesson, but actually during the times that the stress is at its greatest. It is possible to apply the technique to any situation in your life. Actors, musicians and performers of all kinds have found the Alexander Technique to be very beneficial, because to perform in front of an audience is to put the mind and body into a very stressful situation, and a performer will often respond to this stress by misusing the body in a very extreme way, as Alexander was the first to discover when he lost his voice during public recitals.

It was no accident that Alexander was a performer. If he hadn't been, his voice problem, which was a result of his extreme misuse on stage, might never have developed. But the misuse would still have been there, since misuse during performance is usually an exaggeration of our everyday misuse. If Alexander had not been an actor and had not developed his technique in order to cure his voice problem, he might well have developed neck or back pain or some other malfunctioning symptom as he grew older, as a result of his habitual misuse. Fortunately for us he *was* an actor, who found the solution to his voice problems by studying his misuse of himself, and then teaching his discoveries to others.

• *Observing Your Use* •

As you read this book, pause for a moment, and begin to give attention to the position you are in. Is your back straight or bent, and if bent in what way? What is happening to your abdomen, is it compressed? What is happening to your shoulders? Is your head on one side? If you are sitting, are your feet touching the floor? Where are your legs and arms? What is the expression on your face? For example, do you tend to frown, or raise your eyebrows when you read? Have you been in this position for quite a long time? Is it beginning to feel fixed and stiff? Do you notice other sensations in your body? These are all observations about how you are using your self while reading. Please don't make assumptions at this stage about what is good use and what is misuse. These will be explained later in the book. For now, simply observe what is going on with curiosity, but without judgement. If you are feeling fixed and stiff, take a few moments to stretch and move around however you wish, all the time giving your attention to the way in which you are moving. I am not asking you to try to do it 'right', just to notice what is going on, giving your attention to your bodily movements.

The Whole Self

Our use involves the positions we put our bodies in and the movements that we make getting from one position to another. But the way in which we use our selves is not restricted to the way in which we use our bodies. Alexander was concerned with the whole self, and how we use it. Our thoughts and feelings play as great a part in our use as do our physical movements. In fact they are inseparable. The mental decision to do even the simplest activity, such as walking, sitting, or standing, precedes and is maintained during that activity. Alexander called this psychophysical unity. He demonstrated that every 'physical' activity has a mental component, and vice versa. What we are thinking and feeling when we sit, stand, wash the dishes or drive a car is going to affect the way in which we do it enormously. And this is even more true for stressful situations, such as taking examinations or performing in front of an audience.

• *Observing Your Whole Self* •

If you now add to your observations about how you are using your body, observations about the thoughts and feelings you are having as you read this book, you will be getting more information about your use. For some people the reading will feel like a treat and for others it will feel like a chore. Some people will be thinking in agreement with me and other people will be having very critical thoughts. And the person who finds the reading a treat may also be the person who is highly critical of what she is reading. And in addition to thoughts about the book there are probably lots of other thoughts popping into your mind which you may notice. Our mental and emotional responses are complex and unique to each one of us. What do you observe about your mental and emotional responses? In particular, notice your reaction to being asked to stop and observe what you are doing, sensing, thinking and feeling. Is this easy for you or does it fill you with irritation and resistance?

Habitual Use

The false poise and carriage of the body, the incorrect and laboured habits of breathing that are the cause of many troubles besides the obvious ill-effects on the lungs and heart, the degeneration of the muscular system, the partial failure of many vital organs, the morbid fatty conditions that destroy the semblance of men and women to human beings – all these things and many more that combine to cause debility, diseases and death are the result of incorrect habits of mind and body, all of which may be changed into correct and beneficial habits if once we can clear away that first impeding habit of thought which stands between us and conscious control. (FMA, *MSI*)

Much of our behaviour is governed by habit. It would be impossible to survive if we did not have the ability to operate automatically, responding to stimuli in a learned habitual way. If you have ever learned to drive a car, or ride a bicycle, you will probably have experienced how something that seemed impossibly difficult and complex initially, changes into an easy habitual activity.

Developing habits is an essential part of the way in which we learn new skills. Habitual behaviour is something we do *without having consciously to think about it*, or with a minimum of attention, and this allows our minds to give attention to other matters. For example, having learned how to stand as a child, as an adult it is fairly easy to stand and read a newspaper at the same time, and so our behaviour becomes more complex. This is fine if we learned our skills in a way that is beneficial to us, but it is a big stumbling block when we want to change the way we are operating in our lives. Because in order to change, first of all, *we have once again to start consciously thinking about how we are doing something*, and then we come up against the power of our habits, for even giving attention to our behaviour is contrary to habit. It can be very difficult to undo learned and habitual behaviour, and learning how to do this is a large part of what the Alexander Technique teaches. If it seems difficult to go back into that conscious awareness of how to drive a car, or ride a bicycle, then how much more difficult to unlearn habitual behaviour that was learned in our infancy, like sitting, standing, walking or talking. But if we wish to improve the use of the self, then unlearning these old habits is what needs to happen. And before we can unlearn them we need to find out exactly what they are. As the story of this book unfolds it will become clearer what to look for when you observe your use, what Alexander meant by good use and misuse of the self. Beginning by observing oneself carefully, noticing how you do things without any concept of good and bad, is one of the first skills involved in the art of changing.

• *Getting to Know Your Habits* •

You have already had a chance to pause and observe how you are using your mind and body while reading this book. From now on, start giving some conscious attention to your use, how you are doing all those many activities that make up your life. Every so often during the day pause and notice what you feel is happening in your mind and body. Start to be aware of habitual behaviour, not just physical habits, but mental and emotional habits too. I would recommend that you keep a notebook in which you make all these observations, as this is one way in which you can notice the changes you are making as you proceed with this work.

It is entirely up to you how much time you give to this process of self-observation. As this activity is probably not habitual for you, it will be interesting to see how difficult you find it to incorporate this non-habitual behaviour of observing yourself into your life. It only requires a few seconds or minutes, every so often, and it is likely that if you turn this into a chore, then that is another of your habitual tendencies, or if you forget to do it, that is another. A sense of humour about oneself is helpful when one begins this journey into self-awareness, but that may not be your habit! Observe yourself as though you are some strange creature from another planet whose behaviour you find utterly fascinating. If you can cultivate that (probably non-habitual) attitude you will find this work the more enjoyable.

Below is a list of activities you may like to observe in yourself. This list could go on endlessly, so I shall just suggest a few things, but I hope you will be looking for other types of habitual behaviour, in addition to my suggestions. It is better that you give attention to these activities every so often throughout the day, rather than putting aside a special time for them, because then you are developing a new habit of being self-aware as you live your life, and as you practise this you will learn much more about yourself and how you use yourself than if you create an unreal practice situation in which to observe yourself.

Standing — When you are standing, for instance in a queue, where does the weight of your body fall? Do you tend to stand on one leg, and if so which leg? Is it always the same one? Does the weight tend to fall through the front or the back of the foot, or is it distributed more to the outside or the inside of the foot. What sensations do you experience in your feet? What do you do with your head when standing? Does it tend to lean over to one side? Notice what you do with your arms and hands, your shoulders and chest, your pelvis. Notice any sensations you may be feeling in your body. (*Fig. 1.1*)

Fig. 1.1

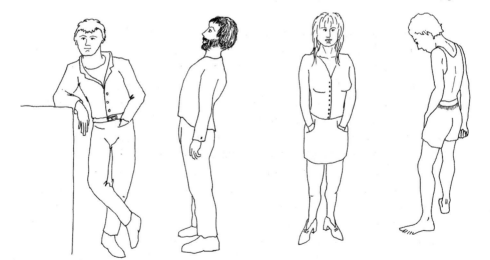

Different ways of standing

Sitting — In a similar way, observe where the weight falls when you are sitting, and give attention to that sensation. Do you carry the weight more on one buttock? What do you do with your legs when sitting? Do your feet touch the floor? What do you do with your head? Also notice if your back is curved or straight, and whether your shoulders are hunched or dropped, or go backwards or forwards. Notice any sensations that you become aware of as you turn your attention onto your self. Build up a picture of your body in the sitting position. (*Fig. 1.2*)

Fig. 1.2

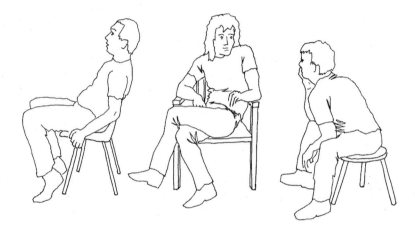

Different ways of sitting

Walking — This time you are observing yourself while moving, which is more complex. Once again notice where the weight lands on your feet. Build up a moving picture of yourself walking. Do you have a sense that one part of your body is leading you when you walk, for example your pelvis, or your chest, or some other part? Notice other people walking and see if it looks as though they are being led by a certain part of the body. Look at the differences in the way different people walk (or stand, or sit). How does your walk alter when you are tired, or full of energy, happy or sad? And notice your thoughts and feelings. Does walking become associated with habitual thoughts or emotions?

Talking — First of all try talking to yourself, and do it somewhere where no-one is going to be watching, such as in the bathroom. This is useful because you can use the mirror to help your observations. To begin with do not use the mirror. Start talking about something quite simple, such as what you are planning to do that day, and give attention to your whole self, not just the face and throat, in the way I have described in the 'Standing' section. Then give attention to your head and neck, your mouth, chin and jaw, your eyes. Notice what you do with your hands and feet when you are talking, and with the rest of your body. Is there some particular part of you that seems to get very tense when you talk? Do you notice other sensations anywhere?

Now observe yourself in the mirror, as you talk. See where the muscles are working in your face, throat and shoulders. Notice also the thoughts and feelings you are having as you do this exercise, especially your responses to looking in the mirror. There should be a great wealth of habitual responses for you to find in there!

After examining yourself talking on your own, see how easy or difficult it is for you to observe yourself when you are talking to someone else. Remember you are looking for an idea or a picture of what your body is doing, the sensations it is feeling, as well as the habitual thoughts and emotions you may notice cropping up when you talk, such as 'I do enjoy communicating', or 'I hate the sound of my voice/accent/lisp' etc..

The ring of the telephone, or the doorbell — Notice your immediate reaction to this stimulus and what your habitual response is to the telephone and/or the doorbell ringing. Notice not only what you do but also what you think and feel.

Waking up — What are the first sensations, thoughts and feelings you have when you wake up. What position are you in? Is it the same every morning?

Later on Pooh and Piglet walked home thoughtfully together in the golden evening, and for a long time they were silent.

'When you wake up in the morning, Pooh,' said Piglet at last, 'what's the first thing you say to yourself?'

'What's for breakfast?' said Pooh. 'What do you say, Piglet?'

'I say, I wonder what's going to happen exciting today?' said Piglet.

Pooh nodded thoughtfully. 'It's the same thing,' he said.

A.A. Milne, *Winnie the Pooh*

Chapter Two

The Semi-Supine Habit

But in the first place it is essential to understand the difference between the habit that is recognized and understood and the habit that is not. The difference . . . is that the first can be altered at will and the second cannot. (FMA, *MSI*)

I have talked about the necessities of habits and the dangers of them. As we learn to develop more conscious awareness in our lives then we can operate more from choice and less from habit. But that does not mean that we lose the skill of operating habit-ually, or automatically. We become able to choose our habits, ones that will be help-ful and beneficial to us, so that we begin to rule them rather than allowing them to rule us. One new habit I have already mentioned as being a good one to cultivate is the habit of self-observation. The more you can give attention to your use, until it becomes automatic and you don't have to remind yourself to be aware, the better. As we develop the theory of the Alexander Technique in later chapters you will become clearer as to what to look for in your use, but it is still valuable to be giving attention now to how you are doing things. I would like to introduce another wonderful new habit into your lives. This is the habit of lying down in the semi-supine position for about twenty minutes to half an hour. If possible you should do this twice a day, (or more if you wish), once round about midday and the other time at about six o'clock, about the time when a lot of people are arriving home from work. In this way the day is broken up into periods when you take your body out of the vertical and into the horizontal plane for a short time. You lie in a position of maximum rest for the spine, during which a powerful rejuvenating process can occur.

• *Getting Into The Semi-Supine Position* •

The position I want you to lie in is shown in figure 2.6. I would like you to get into this position with care. Have a look at the sequence of pictures showing how to get into the final semi-supine position, (*Figs. 2.1 – 2.6*). Don't rush into this position because the way you lie down will either help or hinder the process of lying down.

If you get down in a very tense way then you may spend all your lying down time unravelling the tensions that you got yourself into while lying down. First of all read through all the instructions below, and then read through the instructions for lying down, again, before attempting to do it. Remember you are beginning a new process, and it is concerned with the way in which you do things, so it doesn't matter how long it takes for you to work out how to lie down. We are not concerned with the achievement of lying down but with the process of it.

Be sure the room and floor are warm enough for you to lie down. If they are not you may need to put more rugs under you and a rug over you to keep you warm. Coldness creates muscle tension, so it is important not to let yourself get cold when you are lying down. Also it will help if the clothes you are wearing are not too tight, so your legs can feel quite free with the knees bent up, and your breathing is not restricted by your clothing in any way.

As you can see from the picture, you are going to be lying with your head resting on paperback books. Some people need only one or two books, and other people need eight or more medium sized paperbacks. To get a rough idea of how many books you will need stand against a wall with your bottom and shoulder blades touching the wall. (*Fig. 2.1*) Stand as you would normally stand if there weren't a wall there. Now measure with your fingers the space between your head and the wall. Add an inch to this measurement and this will give you the depth of paperback books that you need. If you are having Alexander lessons your teacher will help you find the exact height of the books for your personal head-neck relationship, taking into account that it may change because you are changing.

1. Place the number of books that you estimate you require on the carpet or rug, with a few extra books close by. Stand about four or five feet away from the books at the other end of the rug, facing away from the books. Be aware of your body standing, neither tense nor collapsed, and be aware of the weight of your body passing through your feet, and that there is an equal and opposite force rising up through your body, and out through the top of your head, (*Fig. 2.1*)

2. Go down on one knee, and then onto two knees, (*Fig. 2.2 - 2.3*). Then sit down and bring your feet up close to your bottom. Check that your books are roughly in the right place if you now roll down onto them, and if they are not, move your bottom in line with the books. Move your bottom towards your feet, so that bottom

Fig. 2.1

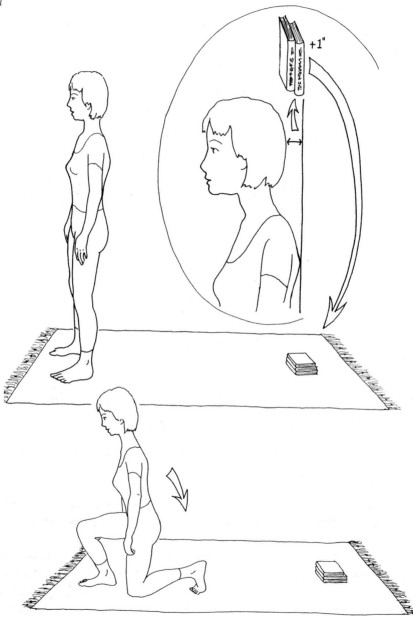

Fig. 2.2

Fig. 2.3

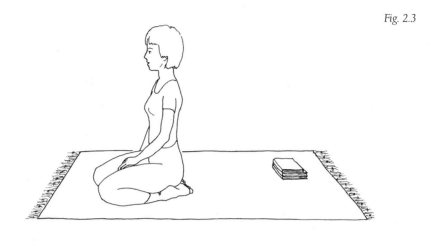

Fig. 2.4

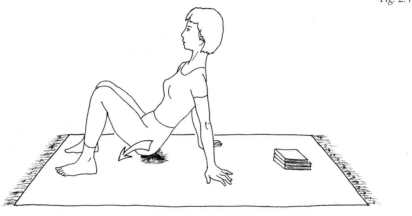

and feet are about six to twelve inches apart. By moving your bottom towards your feet you are allowing the lower back to be as open as possible, before rolling down flat. (*Fig. 2.4*)

These instructions may seem very complicated at first, so if you find yourself getting anxious about 'doing it right', just stop and allow yourself to calm down. It doesn't matter if you don't get it right first time. You can see the final picture of how you want to end up, and so make the experience of getting there an enjoyable experiment, not an anxious one.

Fig. 2.5

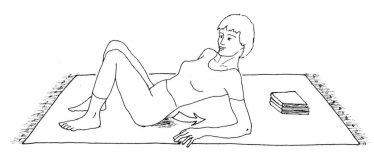

Fig. 2.6

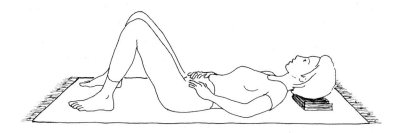

3. Taking your time, lower yourself down onto your elbows, letting the back be loose and relaxed, not held tightly up or down. (Fig. 2.5)

4. Continue to lower your body until your head is resting on the books. Don't worry if you miss the books. Take your head with one hand and lift it up letting the hand take all the weight of the head. By holding your head with your hand you avoid tightening too much in the front of the neck. With the other hand check that the books are in the right place for your head. Now lower your head down onto the books. (Fig. 2.6)

5. It is probable that the position of your head will feel very strange, and may be uncomfortable, because it is not what you are used to. You should be experiencing a gentle lengthening stretch up the back of the neck, which will make your head feel rotated forwards more than usual. Only reduce the number of books if

your head is rotated so far forwards that it is pushing on the larynx in front and making it difficult for you to speak or swallow. If you have very rounded shoulders you may need more books.

6. Now you are lying down, place your hands on your abdomen so they are not touching each other. Your knees should be about hip-width apart, and balanced in such a way that you do not have to tighten your leg muscles for them to stay bent up in this way. Your feet should be quite close to your bottom, about a foot away. If the legs keep falling inwards or outwards adjust the position of the feet, while keeping the knees hip-width apart, until you find a position that feels comfortable, (*Fig. 2.6*)

If the first time you lie down like this you spend most of the time working out how to lie down, whether you are warm enough, how many books you need, how to support your legs, and how to stand up again, then your time will be well spent, because you are taking care of the way in which you begin this new habit in your life. It may take some time to work out the best arrangement of rugs, books and position.

• *Lying Down in Semi-Supine* •

At this point you may like to use side one of the audio cassette tape which accompanies this book, and gives you suggestions for thinking and observing when lying down. If you do not have the tape, I will outline these ideas below.

When you are lying down in the semi-supine position, you are in the position of maximum rest for the spine. This is because by having your knees bent up you allow the curve of the lower back to open out and extend, and similarly with your head on books you allow the curve of the neck to experience a gentle passive stretch. The curves of the spine tend to become over-compressed due to the way we use ourselves. (*Fig. 2.7*). The wear and tear on our spines is enormous and we need to find ways of taking care of this central column of our organism.

Scientific experiments have shown that the human spine degenerates much more rapidly than the rest of us, so that on average it can be said to be twenty years older than the rest of the body. In this light, the Alexander Technique can be seen to be of evolutionary significance, because it teaches a person how to operate well in the upright, so that the spine lengthens upwards rather than collapsing downwards.

Fig. 2.7

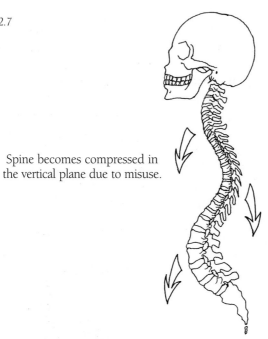

Spine becomes compressed in
the vertical plane due to misuse.

Spine lengthens and releases
in the horizontal plane.

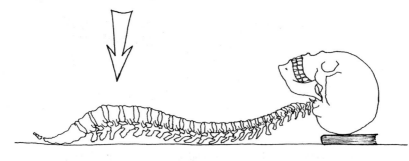

Lying down like this is the best way to start changing the process of deterioration and beginning a process of rejuven-ation. And it is paradoxical but very
important to notice that we start the changing process by stopping. We don't
begin sorting out our problems by doing this, that, or the other, but by stopping
the doing, by saying 'No' to the habitual activities of the day, creating a resting
space for the body, and placing the body in this position of maximum rest for the

spine. So be aware that you are doing something very important towards changing yourself, just by creating the space to lie down in this way and do nothing.

It is possible to use the time when you are lying down in a way that is very beneficial to your whole self, by thinking about your mind and body in certain ways, which I will describe later in the book. But even if you lie down in this position and don't think about your body at all you will be doing it a lot of good. Even if you play music and forget about what's happening to your body as you lie down, there will be muscular releases; the curves of the spine will start to open out, and the discs in between the vertebrae, which are like little sponges which get compressed through misuse, will be able to soak up body fluid and expand and become much more elastic. All this will happen in twenty minutes to half an hour, simply by lying down and allowing the body to sort itself out. (*Fig. 2.8*)

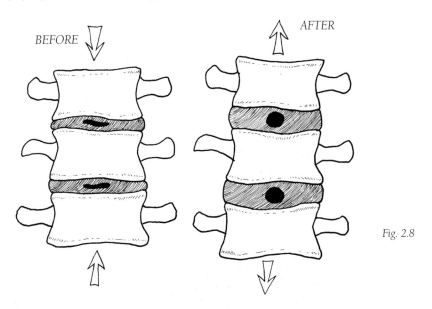

Fig. 2.8

Intervertebral Discs before and after lying in Semi-Supine

• *From 'Doing' to 'Being'* •

First of all, be aware that you are bringing your body into stillness. Notice the sensations that occur as your body settles into this position. Don't keep wriggling about and rearranging yourself. Once you feel you have found a comfortable position, allow yourself to stay like that and become an observer to what is happening in your body and your mind. You are giving yourself permission to take a look at yourself and see what's going on, mentally, emotionally, and physically. You are becoming the listener, listening to the sensations, thoughts and feelings inside your body, and also listening to the sounds and light changes and vibrations that you may notice going on around you on the outside of your body. Notice the thoughts that pass through your consciousness. Don't comment, just observe with interest the kind of thoughts you are having and the speed with which you move from one thought to another. Let a part of you be observing your own thinking and feeling process. Your attention is inwards and outwards, listening.

It is significant that the mechanism with which we listen, and the mechanism with which we balance our bodies are both located in the ear. There is an important connection between listening and balance, and as you move into this listening, attentive mode notice how this affects the quality of your experience, the quality of the sensations, emotions and thoughts. So much of our lives we are 'actors', busily 'doing' one thing or another, but by lying down like this we become 'observers', aware of the process of 'being' rather than 'doing'. We are changing an important habit, and this may be difficult to do. You may find yourself becoming impatient, irritable and restless, when you lie down. Remain the observer and notice these responses in yourself. You are learning a lot by watching how you respond to this non-habitual behaviour. On the other hand you may find yourself getting very, very still, and even falling asleep. This also is valuable information for you, about the way you are coping with your life. Every single thing you notice is valuable. Don't judge some things as negative and others as positive. Everything you notice is information about you, a way of getting to know yourself, honestly and without judgement. In order to change we have to know what we want to change. We have to know and accept our own selves as we really are, not as we pretend to be.

You could easily spend the whole period of lying down watching yourself in the way I have suggested, noticing if the quality of sensations, emotions and thoughts change as the body becomes more still. Allow yourself as much time as you wish to do this, and as many times as you wish. Don't hurry yourself to do the next bits of the exercise. All these suggestions are for you to play with in the many times you lie down. You don't have to do them all every time. The more interested and varied you make your lying down process each day the more readily it will become an enjoyable habit.

• *Floor Contact Awareness* •

The back of our body is a part of us that gets very little attention. When we relate to other people we do so to the front of them, and when we look at ourselves in the mirror we look at the front part of ourselves. This is very different for a four-legged animal such as a cat or a dog. A large part of what we see then is the back part of the animal, and the front part is concealed. The lack of attention and awareness we give our backs is matched by the tendency for our backs to be weak. So it is useful when lying down to build up a picture of your back, especially as it is receiving a strong stimulus from the support of the floor.

Notice where your body contacts the floor, and your head contacts the books. Go through all the parts of your body that are in contact with the floor, and get a feeling of that contact. Imagine that the floor is a white sheet of paper and you are covered in paint. Work out what the impression made by your head, your elbows, your feet, your shoulder blades, your pelvis and the rest of your back, would look like upon this white sheet. Notice if the impressions of the right and left foot are different, and whereabouts on the foot the weight lies, front or back, inside or outside, and similarly for the elbows, shoulder blades and different sides of the back and head. In everyday life these parts of your body get very little attention, so try to develop an awareness of them. They really are parts of you, which have probably been very neglected, but from now on you will be getting to know them better and better. When you get up after this mental exercise, try to carry in your mind the picture of the back you have built up.

• *Bodyscan* •

Now begin a scan of the body, giving your attention to the left foot, the toes, the bottom of the foot, the top of the foot and then the left ankle. Do the same for the right foot, and ankle. Now put your attention onto your lower leg, first one leg then the other, then the knees, then the upper legs and hips. Don't do anything, just give attention to that part of your body, as though you were listening to it. Notice what sensations, images and feelings occur as you become aware of different parts of your body. It's often quite revealing to ask different parts of the body how they are, and whether they have anything to say. One student discovered his legs were very angry because he didn't wear clothes that would keep them warm, he neglected them constantly, and then expected them to cycle long distances

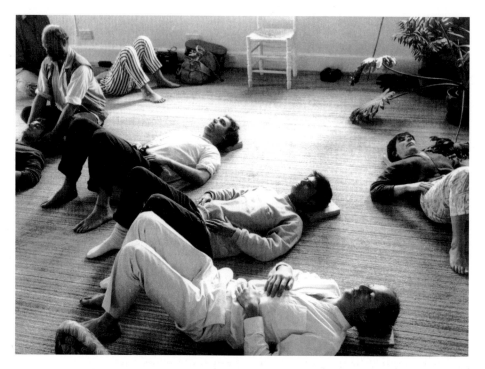

Group work – semi-supine

when they were cold and stiff. I remember my legs being unhappy because they wanted to dance and I led far too sedentary a life for them.

Now give your attention in a similar way to your arms, comparing one arm with the other, the fingers, thumbs, hands, wrists, lower arms, elbows, upper arms and shoulders. Notice the contact of your hand on your abdomen, and how that feels both in the hand and in the abdomen.

Now move your attention to your head. Notice where it contacts the books, and then give your awareness to all the part of the head covered with hair. What does it feel like to have hair on your head? Then see if you can feel your ears, and build up a picture of them. Travel right round the ear. Notice if there is tension in the ear or in the skin around the ear. Similarly observe the forehead, the eyebrows, the eyes, the nose, the cheeks, the lips, the chin, the jaw. Once again you can ask any part of your body to talk to you or to give you an image of itself. Go inside the mouth and give attention to the tongue and the teeth. Notice the breath passing over your upper lip and in and out of your nostrils. Then move your attention onto your neck, the back, the front and sides of it. Feel how the breath affects your neck and also your chest and the trunk of your body. A body scan can take anything from ten minutes to several hours or even days; there is so much material for observation. I am not suggesting you lie down for that length of time to do it, but you may decide you want to spend each session scanning in depth a part of your anatomy.

Just watch your breathing. Don't try to make it long or deep. Get to know it how it really is, without any interference from you based on how you think it should be. And so continue to move your attention onto your shoulders and ribs and chest and down onto your abdomen and pelvis, under the pelvic floor and onto your buttocks, your lower back, your middle and upper back. Then be aware of the sides of your body as well as the back and the front. Scan inside the body, feeling the sensations of your spine rising up through the centre of your body, and all the organs around it like the heart, stomach, liver and intestines, in as much detail as you are able.

Allow this body scanning to be your own creative process. Follow your own routes around the body; do not stick rigidly to the suggestions I have made, but add your own ideas to them. Talk to any parts of your body that you wish to. Notice the parts that you neglect or forget about.

• *Visualization of the Body's Processes* •

The body scanning can be developed further, for those of you who have some knowledge of anatomy and physiology. This time you will be using visualization, rather than noticing sensations, images and thoughts arising from the body, so it is rather different. You can imagine the skeleton inside the body, with all the muscles attached to it, or you can imagine the blood circulating, or the digestive process at work, or the activity of the glands and the lymphatic system. I am not going to go into these here, but offer them as possibilities for you to work with if you wish. If you find it difficult to visualize, then just stay with the kinaesthetic information you are receiving, when you give attention to those areas.

• *Drawing Your Skeleton* •

Without consulting any anatomy books, spend one of your lying-down sessions visualizing your skeleton. As you scan your body, picture just what the skeleton looks like from the tips of your toes to the tips of the fingers and the top of your head. When you get up, draw your visualized skeleton, and only then compare it to the illustration on page 108. Notice which bits you felt better about drawing and whether the bits you got wrong are bits of yourself that you tend to neglect.

• *Getting up from Semi-Supine* •

Getting up from the lying down position should also be done carefully. (See *Figs. 2.9 – 2.14*). While you have been lying down you will have allowed a lengthening and widening of the front and back of you, and if you now raise your head up (the reverse of the way you got down) you will be pulling tight all those muscles in the front of your body that have been releasing as you were lying down. So in order to get up with the least interference to those good changes that have occurred, it is best to roll over sideways. Begin by looking at which side you want to roll over onto, and then let your head follow your eyes, rolling over to the side you have chosen, then let your body follow your head, rolling over onto the side.

Be aware of the quality in your torso while lying down and try to maintain that quality as you roll over onto your side; then use your arms and legs to move into a crawling position. You may like to crawl around the room slowly for a few moments, feeling the contact of your hands and feet with the floor, and the gentle change in your body from stillness into movement. From the crawling position sit back on your heels and then, thinking of the head leading, go into an upwards kneeling position, and from this position stand up. Keep thinking of your back and front being nicely lengthened and widened, and of the weight as you stand being distributed evenly between the inside and the outside of your feet, with very slightly more weight on the heels of the feet than on the front of the feet. Stand quietly for a few moments just noticing how your body feels, especially your neglected back, having rested for half an hour, and then start gently walking around keeping an awareness of your body as you go into the rest of your daily activities. If you are able to keep a notebook and make a record of the things you notice and experience when lying down in this way it will help you keep in touch with the changes taking place in yourself.

I would recommend that you lie down in this position twice a day or more, but if it is impossible for you to do so during the middle of the day then do it as soon as you get back from work. If you are brave enough to cope with the comments, lie down in your work place. I can assure you that more and more people are lying down in their lunch breaks at their places of work. It's even becoming the trendy thing to do! I've

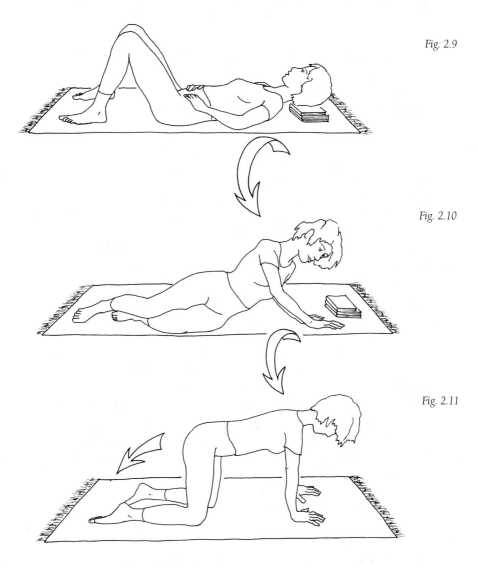

Fig. 2.9

Fig. 2.10

Fig. 2.11

Getting up from the Semi Supine position

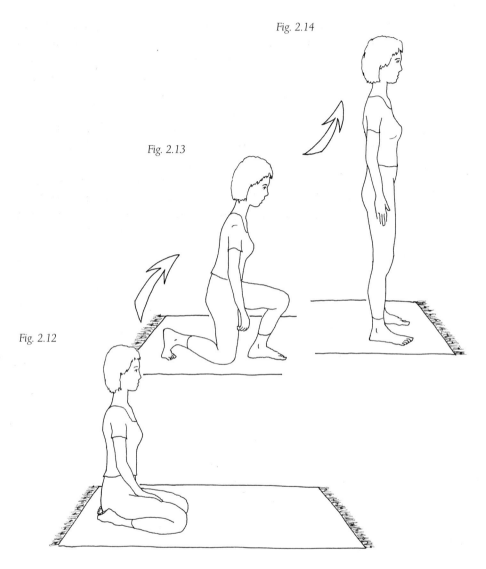

Fig. 2.14

Fig. 2.13

Fig. 2.12

Getting up from the Semi-Supine position

seen someone do it in the middle of a television play on set, and when I worked in the theatre and in television I did it off stage and off set all the time I could. It seems odd that it's acceptable to have a break from work in which you drink a nervous stimulant such as tea or coffee, which will only make you more tired in the long run, whereas it's not acceptable to lie down in semi-supine, and give yourself a real rest, one that genuinely refreshes you. Those people living in warmer countries who take siestas in the middle of the day are doing their bodies much more good than we are. The more we can introduce simple and effective aids to our well-being, like the semi-supine habit, the better. But if you do find yourself the subject of ridicule, notice how that affects you too. If you courageously lie down on your office floor with your stomach in a terrible knot and your mind anxiously preparing itself for defence when the comments come, it's unlikely the lying down will be doing you much good. We are all unique and what may be easy for one person may be torment for another. The whole purpose of this development of self observation is to understand what your individual and unique responses are, and to accept the truth of those responses for you. Only when you really understand your own starting place can you hope to know how to make the next move.

Chapter Three

The Evidence of the Senses

It seems strange to me that although man has thought it necessary in the course of his development in civilization to cultivate the potentialities of what he calls 'mind', 'soul', and 'body', he has not so far seen the need for maintaining in satisfactory condition the functioning of the sensory processes through which these potentialities manifest themselves. (FMA, *UOS*)

In the first two chapters you began the process of developing self-awareness, through observing some of your habits and by creating a space in which you could lie down in semi-supine and give attention to your mind and body. By self-awareness I mean an awareness of many aspects of our internal experience, including thoughts and images, emotions and sensations.

In this chapter I am going to focus more upon the awareness we have of our sensations. Aristotle handed down to us the tradition of the five senses of touch, taste, smell, sight and hearing. All these senses give us information about the outer world. He did not postulate the senses we have which give us information about our inner worlds and it is significant that the study of these is a relatively recent development. Our neglect of this aspect of ourselves is reflected in the way we, in the Western world, have misused our bodies. We are literally 'out of touch' with them, to the extent that physical stress symptoms like backache have now reached serious epidemic proportions. If we had developed a more refined sensory apparatus we would probably have known how to avoid the problems that now beset us in the complex, polluted, and stressful environment in which we struggle to survive.

• *Stimulating a Sensory Awareness through Touch* •

Sit comfortably and take hold of your left foot. Start to stroke the foot and ankle very, very gently as though it were a delicate creature that needed lots of love and attention. Then stroke it more firmly for several seconds. Then massage the foot quite strongly, moving the foot around the ankle joint in as many ways as you can. Finally slap the foot and ankle quite hard with sharp smacks. Repeat this process with the lower leg and the knee joint, and then with the upper leg and hip joint. Take your time about doing this, giving your left leg all the care and attention you can.

Now stand up and feel the sensory difference between the two legs. Slowly walk around noticing the differences in sensory information you receive from the two legs. There will probably be such an enormous difference you will need to give your right leg the same treatment to balance things up.

By stimulating the muscles, the skin and the circulation of the left leg, and by giving the leg lots of mental and emotional attention, through the various types of massage, you really livened up the sensory mechanism of that part of your body. Then you can see how unawake the sensory mechanism tends to be, by comparison with the right leg which probably feels quite dead. If we give more attention to the sensory information available to us, the experience of our bodies, and therefore of being alive, becomes much richer.

In order to have an idea of how we are using our bodies, we make use of a sixth sense that we all have. Called the kinaesthetic sense, it is an important part of our sensory mechanism. Kinaesthesis means 'sensation of muscular effort that accompanies a voluntary motion of the body', and so the kinaesthetic sense gives us an awareness of our movement.

• Using Your Kinaesthetic Sense •

Read the following instructions carefully and then carry them out.

Close your eyes. Now move your arm slowly up above your head with the hand pointing vertically up towards the ceiling. Observe the sensations involved that make it possible for you to move the arm to a particular position without the help of your visual sense. Open your eyes and check that your arm is in the position I suggested.

Close your eyes again. Now move the arm out to the side in line with the shoulder. Once again be aware of the sensations you experience that make it possible for you to know just where to move your arm. Open your eyes and check that your arm is in the position I suggested.

Your ability to know the movement and position of your arm, without using your visual sense, comes from the information of this sixth sense, the kinaesthetic sense, which allows us to know all sorts of things about our use without having to look and see what we are doing. You may have noticed as you moved your arm with your eyes closed, how unusual it is to give any attention to these kinaesthetic sensations upon which we are so very dependent for our co-ordination and well-being. Below is another practical experiment to allow you to explore this more.

Read the instructions carefully and then carry them out.

Close your eyes. Very slowly move one arm up and down and out to the side, exploring the movement of the shoulders, elbows, wrists and fingers, and giving all your attention to those kinaesthetic sensations that accompany movement. Now move the other arm. Experience as fully as you can the sensations involved. Now move your head around and feel the movement of the head on the neck; then move the trunk of your body in different ways; and then experiment with movements of the legs. Experience the sensations of your body from the inside, moving slowly and exploring gently your range of possible movement.

Our kinaesthetic awareness is an awareness of certain sensations that give us information about posture and movement. Not all our feeling sensations are received through this sense; for example the sensation of touch, either touching or being touched, is a separate neurological function, and similarly when we experience painful or pleasurable sensations they are not received through our kinaesthetic sense. The world of our sensations is rich and varied, but sadly undervalued, and under-used. We do not even have the language to distinguish one type of sensation from another with any degree of subtlety .*

The exercises in Chapter One all involve a kinaesthetic awareness, as well as other types of self-awareness, such as awareness of thoughts and feelings and other sensations. Continue with these investigations into your use with the additional understanding you have gained from exploring your kinaesthetic awareness in this section. Allow yourself to experience the kinaesthetic sensations as fully as you can in all that you do.

*The Chinese, with their long cultural tradition of treating disease by means of acupuncture needles, have a much more highly developed language and experience of sensation than we do. The patient is expected to inform the doctor of the type of sensation experienced when the acupuncture needles enter the flesh, and there are many different shades of meaning available to describe subtly different sensations.

UNRELIABLE SENSORY AWARENESS

The more attention we give to our bodily use, by allowing ourselves to experience our many bodily sensations, the more possible it is to refine our self-awareness and improve our use. However, there are dangers and pitfalls, and the greatest of these is that at the beginning of this process our sensory awareness, having been neglected for so long, is very deficient and unreliable. It is somewhat as though we had been deaf for many years and then began to regain our hearing. Firstly we would only hear the loudest and most obvious sounds, and the sounds would tend to be indistinguishable one from another, as though blurred. Only through time, through experiments and mistakes, and ideally with the help of other people who can hear clearly, would we be able to develop a clarity of hearing once more.

• *How Accurate are the Feelings?* •

Read the instructions carefully and then carry them out. The diagrams on page 43 show you pictorially the positions you will be moving into, so look at these before you begin. For these experiments you will need a full length mirror. (Alternatively this work can be done with two people facing each other, and taking it in turns to give the necessary visual feedback.) It is important when you open your eyes to check your accuracy, that you observe very carefully. Don't cheat yourself in order to be right!

1. Stand in front of the mirror about two feet away from it. *Close your eyes*. Place your feet about one foot apart from each other so they are exactly symmetrical to each other. Stand in a relaxed way, your head square on your shoulders and your shoulders symmetrical to each other, as perfectly square and symmetrical as you can be, facing the mirror, keeping your eyes closed. Notice whether your shoulders feel perfectly symmetrical or not. Does one feel higher, tenser, or more pulled forward than the other? Does your head feel as though it is going straight up, or is it tilted to one side or the other? Nobody is perfectly symmetrical. Can you feel differences between the two sides of your body? Notice what they are. (*Fig. 3.1*)

Don't move as you now open your eyes and check whether your head is straight or slightly tilted or twisted to one side. Remember you are looking for very subtle discrepancies from your 'feeling' information. Check whether your shoulders are as you felt them to be when your eyes were closed or slightly different in some way. Notice whether there is any twist on your shoulders or pelvis which interferes with the squareness of your body relative to the mirror. Then look at your feet to see how precisely symmetrical they are or are not.

2. *Close your eyes*. Now move both arms out to the sides so that they are exactly level with the shoulders and square to the mirror, in symmetry with each other. Notice whether your arms feel the same, or different from each other in some way. Open your eyes and carefully check your accuracy. (*Fig. 3.2*)

3. *Close your eyes* and bend the arms at the elbow, so that the upper arms are level with the shoulders, while the lower arms are exactly vertical, with the hands pointing up towards the ceiling, and so that both hands are symmetrical with each other. Keep your attention on your sensory awareness as you do this. For example, does one arm feel stiffer or in some way different from the other? Now open your eyes and check your accuracy. (*Fig. 3.3*)

4. *Close your eyes* and move your arms so that they are pointing towards the floor at an angle of 45 degrees. Let the arms be exactly symmetrical to each other. Gather your kinaesthetic information and then open your eyes and check your accuracy. (*Fig. 3.4*)

5. Make some more experiments for yourself, along these lines, using different parts of the body in addition to the arms.

6. Sit comfortably on a chair or stool in front of the mirror. Now close your eyes and start to move your head as slowly as you possibly can towards the left. The head should be moving as slowly as the minute hand of a clock, that is, imperceptibly slowly. See how slowly you can do this. Once again it is a very non-habitual activity. When you feel you have moved your head quite a long way and you have an idea of what position you are in, open your eyes and see how accurate you are in your guess. Now move the head back towards the centre and stop at what you feel to be the central position of the head. See how accurate you are. Now repeat the exercise, moving your head to the right.

7. For this experiment you will need two sets of bathroom scales and a friend to read them for you! Stand with one foot on each scale and organize yourself so that

you feel the weight to be balanced on each foot equally. Now ask your friend to read the scales. (This exercise involves more than the kinaesthetic sense, as you are using the sensory information from the pressure on the base of the feet as well. However this is all part of your sensory mechanism as a whole.)

8. Continue making more experiments of your own design, to investigate your sensory accuracy. It is important that when you open your eyes you observe in the minutest detail.

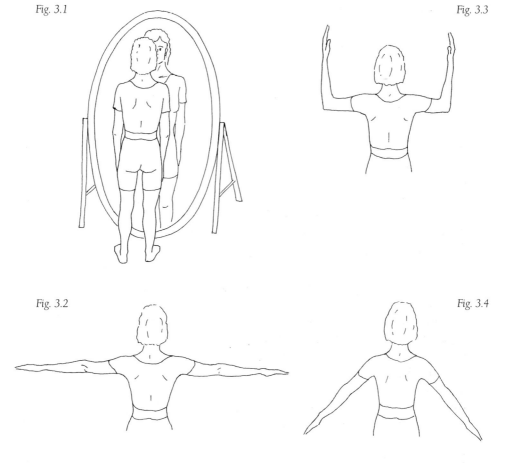

Fig. 3.1

Fig. 3.3

Fig. 3.2

Fig. 3.4

Exploring the kinaesthetic sense

• *Right is Wrong, and Wrong is Right* •

It should be clear from all the above exercises that your sensory mechanism is probably reliable enough to do fairly simple, unsubtle movements, with a satisfactory degree of accuracy, but when you require more refined and subtle information you can be less certain of its accuracy.

One important reason why our kinaesthetic sense is unreliable is because of the power of our habitual behaviour. What is habitual, or 'normal', feels right. And so if we habitually misuse ourselves it will nevertheless feel right to do so and anything different will feel wrong and awkward to begin with. This is one of the biggest stumbling blocks to learning to change the use of ourselves.

If you have spent the last twenty years of your life walking around with your head very slightly tilted to the right, and an Alexander Teacher comes along and straightens the position of the head, it will feel as though the head is tilting to the left. This is because your kinaesthetic sense will be informing you of the movement of the head towards the left away from your 'normal' position which you will assume to be central. Similarly, lots of students lean back from the waist. When this is corrected by a teacher they feel as though they are leaning forward, when in fact they may be standing straight for the first time in many years. The changed position will feel wrong, even though it is an improvement on the position which feels right. And so in order to change you often have to allow yourself to feel wrong, which isn't easy!

Alexander spent a lot of time discussing the poverty of our sensory awareness, which he described in many ways, the most common being 'unreliable sensory appreciation'. He gave many examples of how students were misled by their sensory mechanisms. On one occasion he worked upon a little girl whose spine was severely distorted, to the extent that she was unable to walk. After working on her with his hands, Alexander managed to straighten out the child's body considerably, and certainly to the extent that it was noticeable to the child's parents. When he had finished the little girl said to her mother 'Oh! Mummy, he's pulled me out of shape'. For this child, the norm was in fact to be out of shape, and this felt right. Anything else felt wrong and out of shape. And we all suffer from this paradoxical problem to a greater or lesser degree.

It seems perhaps that what I have given with one hand, in the first chapter, that is the possibility to become aware of your use, I have now taken away with my other hand, in this chapter. Now I am saying that this newly explored awareness is at least faulty if not totally debauched! Alas I have no panacea for this dilemma.

It is one of those terrible facts of life. We need to refine our self-awareness, but the tools with which we must do it are blunt and in need of refinement themselves.

An Alexander teacher is trained to help you refine and improve the reliability of your sensory mechanism. Everybody misuses themselves in different ways, and a teacher can help to point out to the student what is going wrong, and then show how to put that right. Individual attention is important. It is the equivalent of the deaf person getting help from a person with good hearing, for every Alexander Teacher has spent three years in training to refine his own sensory apparatus, and so his sensory appreciation is much more reliable, and this enables him to teach students how to refine their own sensory apparatus, and their self-awareness in general.

Alexander went through this process on his own, without the help of a teacher, which is one example of how he was such a remarkable person. He recognised that his own sensory mechanisms were faulty, and so he used his visual sense. With the help of mirrors he observed himself in minute and subtle detail, discovering what he was doing wrong, how his feelings and his observations were often at odds; and how he could learn to stop doing the wrong thing and learn to do the right thing, which then would develop a reliable sensory awareness, because, after a time, the right thing would also feel right. In this way he monitored his kinaesthetic awareness by means of his visual awareness. His experiments went on for many years. We will look at these later on in this book.

Although our sensory mechanisms tend to be unreliable, I am not suggesting that we should give up on them and ignore them altogether. They are all we have got! The process of developing and refining our sensory appreciation is a slow one, but it can be a fascinating and very enjoyable one. We are like creatures coming out of a long sleep, who need to be treated with care and respect, but also with an awareness that our slumbers have left us short of important skills which now need to be carefully cultivated if we are to survive as a species.

We must give the child of today and of the future, as a fundamental of education, as complete a command of his or her kinaesthetic systems as is possible, so that the highest possible standard of 'free expression' may be given in every sphere of life and in all forms of human activity. We must build up, co-ordinate, and readjust the human machine so that it may be in tune. (FMA, *MSI*)

Chapter Four

How Muscles Work

For when defects in the poise of the body, in the use of the muscular mechanisms, and in the equilibrium are present in the human being, the condition thus evidenced is the result of undue rigidity of parts of the muscular mechanisms associated with undue flaccidity of others.
(FMA,MSI)

There is a lot of misunderstanding in our society today as to what constitutes good muscle tone. Some people point to our athletes as the height of physical well-being, but then others will show how badly athletes suffer as they get older. Joggers have been known to drop dead! Perhaps it would be best to just sit and meditate rather than exercise? Some people go in for body building, thinking the bigger they can make their muscles the better, and therefore supposedly the fitter they will be. There are a lot of false conceptions about what is the optimum state for our muscles, what constitutes good muscle tone, over-active tone (hypertonus), and poor tone (hypotonus).

Operating with good use could be described as doing everything with the minimum possible muscular effort. We want just enough tension in the muscles for them to do what is required at any given moment, no more and no less. 'Maximum output from minimum muscular effort' would be one definition of the most efficient use of the body. And misuse could be explained in terms of too much tension, or too much extension of the muscles, that is the muscles are too tight, too loose, too short or too long.

The Alexander Technique is concerned with our use, with the way in which we move. When an Alexander Teacher places her hands on a student, one of the things she is assessing is the quality of the musculature, whether it be too tight, or too collapsed, whether it feels over-active, balanced, or inert and flaccid. Our muscles are what create movement in the body and so it is helpful to have a basic understanding of how they function. Before I embark on an explanation of muscle function, I must point out that I am only an amateur anatomist, and I want to explain the activity of muscles as simply as I can in a way that can be understood by the non-scientific reader.

Muscles are elastic tissues which, because of their ability to contract and expand,

and also to tighten and release, are responsible for all the movement of the body. There are two quite different kinds of muscles in the body, which perform very different functions. They are called voluntary and involuntary muscles.

Involuntary Muscles

A lot of our muscles contract and expand automatically. These include the heart muscle*, the muscles that line the blood vessels, the stomach and intestines, parts of the eye mechanism, and so on. All the time lots of activity is going on in the body without us doing anything about it. We call these muscles involuntary muscles because they operate without our conscious control. Whatever we are thinking or doing, our heart goes on beating, the blood circulates, the digestive system digests, our eyes adjust to differences in light and focus, and lots of other quite miraculous operations quietly carry on without any intervention from our conscious selves.

Voluntary or Skeletal Muscle

The other kind of muscle is called voluntary muscle because we do have a certain amount of control over its functioning. Although the expanding part of the muscle action is automatic, the contracting part of its action occurs when we decide to do something. We can make our body move, in a way that we can't make our digestive system digest. Nevertheless, Alexander did not like to call these muscles voluntary muscles because we have far less conscious control over their contracting actions than we believe we have, since they are governed by our habitual use. This type of muscle is also called skeletal muscle because it is attached to the bones of the body. Our flesh is composed of hundreds of skeletal muscles, some large, some small.

The Alexander technique is primarily concerned with this type of muscle, in that we want to have a better conscious control over its contracting and expanding functions. We want to be able to stop unnecessary habitual contractions, encourage expansion in chronically contracted muscle, and liveliness in collapsed and overexpanded muscle.

*Anatomists usually put the heart muscle in a category of its own, because although it is an involuntary muscle, it is a little different from all the other involuntary muscles. Because our interest lies mainly with the voluntary muscles, I have included the heart in the 'involuntary' category for the sake of simplicity.

Each skeletal muscle is made up of hundreds and thousands of muscle fibres, which are like long thin elastic threads. Each of these threads or fibres is enclosed by a protective sheath. Bundles of fibres are grouped together inside another fibrous sheath, and these bundles are all contained in a larger fibrous sack. It is this totality that we call the muscle. (*Fig. 4.1*) One end of this sack is connected to one bone and the other end is connected to another bone. When the muscle contracts, as a result of thousands of individual fibres contracting, the bones move, relative to each other, usually causing a joint, such as the shoulder joint, elbow joint etc., to move.

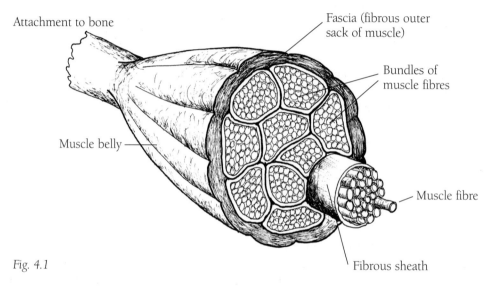

Attachment to bone

Fascia (fibrous outer sack of muscle)

Bundles of muscle fibres

Muscle belly

Muscle fibre

Fibrous sheath

Fig. 4.1

Cross Section of a Muscle Belly

When a muscle contracts, it becomes shorter in length. When it expands it becomes longer. So we also describe a muscle as shortening or lengthening. The action of the muscle is to contract and bring about a movement in the joint. The muscle becomes shorter and pulls the bones together. (*Fig. 4.2*). There is no way this same muscle could push the bones apart by lengthening. The bones can only be moved apart by a different set of muscles shortening.

The muscle contracts because of a stimulus from the nervous system. In the spinal cord of the central nervous system are thousands of nerve cells, called motor neurons. Each of these nerve cells connects to several muscle fibres, by means of a long nerve fibre. (*Fig. 4.3*)

All the muscle fibres connected to a nerve cell respond as a unit when an impulse is transmitted down the nerve fibre. The response is a brief contraction, like a twitch. When a muscle fibre contracts, it shortens by up to half its length. With hundreds of motor neurons transmitting an impulse as often as fifty times per second, and many thousands of muscle fibres responding, the muscle as a whole tenses and shortens. The power of the contraction varies according to the number of motor neurons transmitting an impulse, so the muscle can be very tense and shortened, or less tense, or less shortened, with many fine variations according to the impulses transmitted by the nervous system.

So when we decide to do something, such as walk towards a shelf, raise an arm to reach for something, and lift it down, our decision to make those movements is transmit-

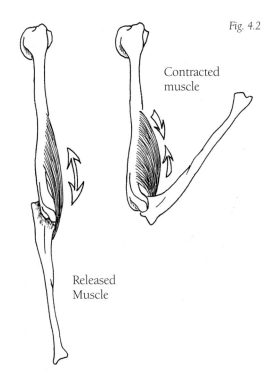

Fig. 4.2

Contracted muscle

Released Muscle

Contraction of the Muscle brings about a Movement in the Joint

ted through the nervous system to the muscles. What is important to note is that our power to control our muscles through action is limited to our ability to make them contract, or shorten. We can do nothing to make a muscle lengthen.

To use an analogy, compare the action of a light switch and a doorbell. With a light switch you have to do something to switch it on, and do something else to switch it off. With a doorbell you do something to switch it on, and you stop doing it to switch it off. Our muscles operate on the doorbell model. Whenever you push the button the bell will ring, and as soon as you stop pushing the button the bell will stop ringing. You don't have to do anything else. With a healthy muscle you switch it on (it shortens and tightens) and then as soon as you stop switching it on, it becomes switched off, (it releases).

What I have just described is the action of a healthy muscle. Unfortunately, in most people of adult age muscles are no longer in such a healthy state. In order to understand what can go wrong with our muscles we need to look a little more at their physiology. As I have already mentioned, muscles consist of an inner and an outer part. The muscle fibre, the meat of the muscle, is surrounded by an outer sack of fibrous tissue. (*Fig 4.1*)

Fig. 4.3

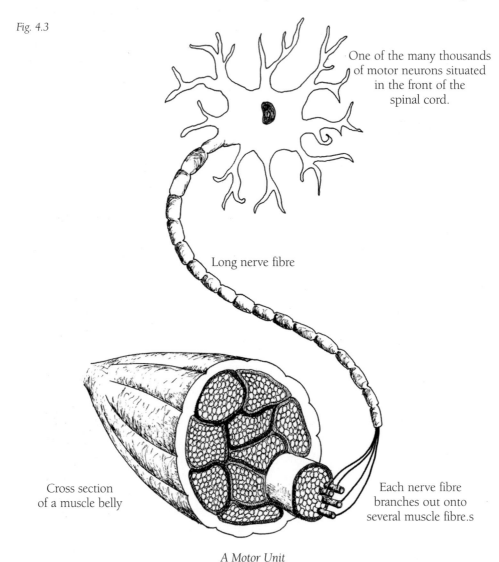

One of the many thousands of motor neurons situated in the front of the spinal cord.

Long nerve fibre

Cross section of a muscle belly

Each nerve fibre branches out onto several muscle fibre.s

A Motor Unit

The Inner Meat of the Muscle

The meat of the muscle is the elastic part which has the ability to shorten or lengthen, and to be tense or to be released. It is the part of the muscle with power to create movement. People often confuse shortening and tension, thinking they are the same; but it is possible to tense a muscle without causing it to move at all, that is without any shortening occurring. An example might be when someone tenses the biceps muscles as a demonstration of strength. This involves tensing the muscle but it does not involve shortening it. The following practical experiment will clarify this.

• *Shortening and Tightening* •

Allow your arm to hang down by your side in a relaxed way. Place the hand of your other arm on the biceps, (*Fig. 4.4*). Now feel the tension when you move your lower arm to the horizontal position, bending the elbow, (*Fig. 4.5*). Now find somewhere you can rest your arm in this position, and allow the muscle to release, (*Fig. 4.6*).

So it is possible for you to move your arm by shortening and tensing the biceps

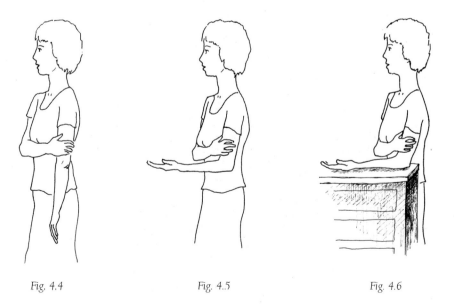

Fig. 4.4   Fig. 4.5   Fig. 4.6

51

muscle, and then for you to release the biceps muscle even though the muscle is still in a shortened state.

Now repeat the above exercise and this time make the muscle work as hard as you can in order to lift the lower arm, and hold the muscle as tense as you can before releasing it. Then repeat the movement using the absolute minimum of muscular tension to perform the action.

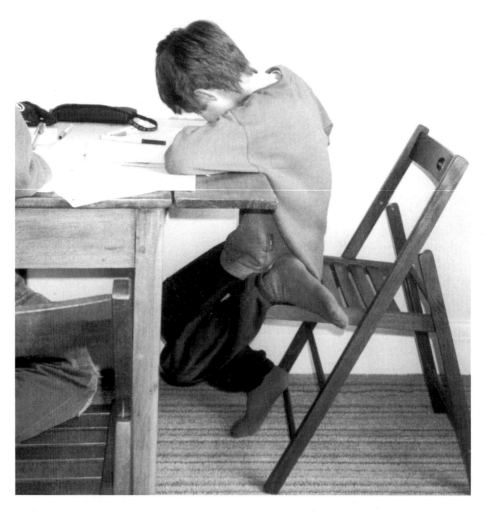

Children are taught how to write but not how to write with good use

One of the objects of the Alexander Technique is to create a state of play in the meat of the muscles so that they only use the minimum necessary tension and shortening for any activity. In our daily lives, many of us use a ridiculous amount of tension to perform the most delicate actions. Handwriting is a good example of this. When you think how light a pen is, and what delicate strokes are required to mark a paper, it is interesting to watch the contortions of the entire body that people often get into when writing. Another example is the playing of a musical instrument. Before I took Alexander lessons my shoulders used to ache with tension after my piano practice. When I learned to release my shoulders I found my piano practice could actually act like a subtle shoulder massage, and my shoulders would often be tingling with delightful releasing sensations after I had been playing for about fifteen minutes.

So in order to improve our use we need to learn to allow the meat of the muscles to be as released as is possible, whatever the situation, whether we are digging the garden, making a speech, writing a letter, or lying down resting. Each of these activities has a different level of appropriate muscle tension. One problem that regularly occurs for many people is that they do some quite strenuous activity like digging the garden, and then are unable to release the muscle tension that was appropriate for that activity, when doing the next activity, such as eating a meal, or reading a book, for which such a high level of muscular tension is quite inappropriate. We also tend to create a lot of muscular tension when we are in an emotionally stressful situation and experiencing a lot of fear and anxiety. Learning to release the muscular tension in these situations is also very important because, if we don't, the fear and anxiety become habitual and we are likely to become 'worriers', fixed in a state of habitual anxiety because of unreleased muscle tension.

The Outer Sack of the Muscle

The sack of the muscle is also able to shorten and lengthen with the action of the meat inside it, but it does not have the elastic power of the meat of the muscle. It is plastic rather than elastic. Its function is to support and protect the meat of the muscle.

If the meat of the muscle has become habitually shortened, the sack will shorten with it and in time will not be able to lengthen to the full stretch of the original healthy muscle. In effect the sack of the muscle shrinks to fit the habitually shortened meat of the muscle. So if the inner meat of the muscle is habitually shortened, or if a person's movement is restricted and limited, the meat of the muscle will slowly lose its freedom as the outer sack tightens up around it.

HEALTHY AND DIS-EASED MUSCLE

Continual readjustment of the parts of the body without undue physical tension is most beneficial, as is proved by the high standard of health and long life of acrobats. It is a significant fact that the very reverse is the case with athletes, showing that undue muscular tension does not conduce to health and longevity. (FMA,MSI)

It is important for the health of the muscle that it experiences a wide range of movement, which prevents shortening in the outer sack of the muscle. It is also important that that movement is accomplished with the minimum shortening and the maximum release in the meat of the muscle. When the muscles are habitually over-contracted and shortened, or habitually over-extended and collapsed, the neuromuscular system loses its liveliness and vibrancy.

If a muscle is in a healthy state it will contract upon demand, and release as soon as that demand is no longer made. It will also extend easily if it is passively stretched by the action (contraction) of other muscles. What I want to stress is that our doing is very good for the creation of muscle contraction, but muscle release occurs automatically; and if for some reason that muscular release will not occur, nothing we do will help it. To return to the analogy of the doorbell, at this point it has become stuck and just keeps on ringing. There are ways of creating muscular release in chronically shortened muscle, but these methods have nothing to do with doing at all.

• *Exploring Some of the Actions of your Hand and Wrist* •

Clench your fist. You have made several muscles contract. Now stop clenching the fist. Don't do anything else, like opening the hand out. Simply stop clenching and feel the tense muscles begin to release. If you now allow your arm and hand to hang down and you swing the arm around gently for a few seconds you will get a sense of how much those muscles will release as a result of gravity acting upon the hand. Allow time for the muscles to release and observe the sensations involved in this process. Some people's hands will be quite open now, other people's will still be quite closed, which shows a certain amount of habitual shortening in those muscles, so they are not able to lengthen and release easily.

If the muscles don't automatically release from the closed position when you let the arm and hand hang down by your side, it is because the demand upon them to contract has been so powerful and continuous the contraction of the muscles has become habitual. Notice how often during the day you close your fist, or whether you make a lot of movements holding the fingers tightly closed.

Now extend the wrist backwards. This involves contracting an opposite set of muscles, and allowing the first set to go through a passive stretch, (*Figs. 4.8 - 4.10*).

Fig. 4.8

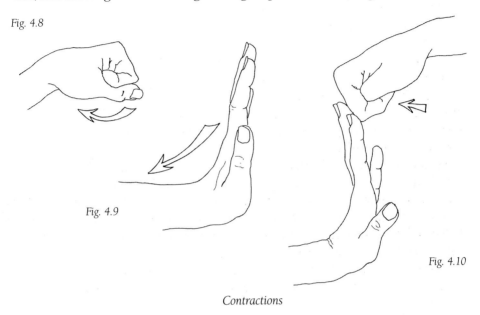

Fig. 4.9

Fig. 4.10

Contractions

It should be possible to extend the hand back almost to a right angle. Now press the fingers backwards gently, as far as they will go, by exerting gentle pressure with the other hand. Stop doing that and see to what position the fingers return, and then see how they respond when you let the arm and hand hang down again.

When you hold the fingers open with the wrist bent back, and then let go, there is no problem about the muscles that pulled the hand back releasing, because this is not a habitual position or activity for the hand. If you found you could not bend back the hand very far, this is probably because the habitually shortened muscles would not allow you to stretch the hand back further. When the muscles become shortened in this way, nothing we do can release them, and this is why vigorous exercise, when a person does not have a good state of muscle tone in the body, can cause pulled muscles or tendons, as many people discover when they go on some sort of exercise programme.

Muscles Balance Each Other

As you may have noticed from the above exercise, we have one set of muscles which can close the hand into a fist, and another set which opens the hand out. We also use the downwards force of gravity to create muscular releases in the body, such as when the hand is hanging down.

Our muscles are organized in balancing sets throughout the body, one set of muscles performing one activity, such as rotating the arm inwards, and another set performing the opposite activity of rotating the arm outwards. One set of muscles will bend the leg at the knee, and another set will straighten the leg outwards. The subtle differences in movement, involving slightly different permutations of muscles for each variation, makes this balancing of muscles very complex, but the general principle holds that our muscles are organized in opposing or antagonistic groups.

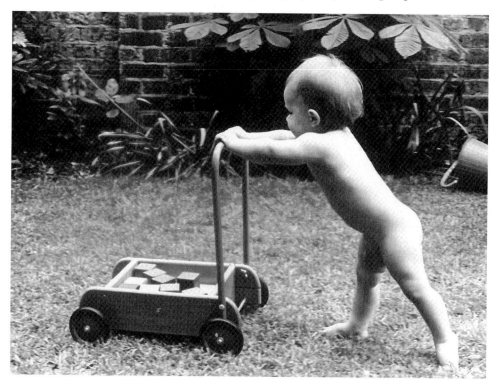

The musculature of this young child is integrated and in balance

• *Working with Antagonistic Groups of Muscles* •

The following suggestions should be carried out gently. They are simply to demonstrate antagonistic movements. Do not do them if they cause you any pain.

THE ARM

Hold your arm in front of you so that you can see
the movements of the hand, wrist and arm.

Fig 4.11

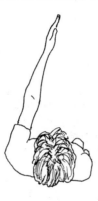

Fig. 4.12

Fig. 4.13

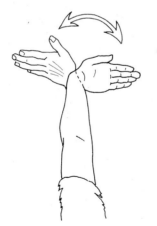

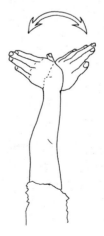

Move the hand inwards and then outwards.   Move the hand from one side to the other.

Fig. 4.14

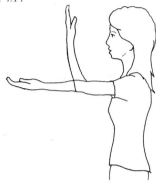

Fig. 4.15

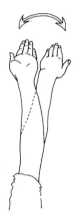

Move the lower arm upwards from
the elbow, and then downwards.

Rotate the lower arm inwards and
then outwards from the elbow.

Fig. 4.16.

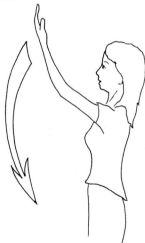

Fig. 4.17

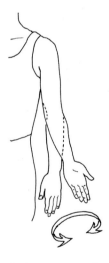

Move the whole arm upwards towards you,
and then downwards. Do this exercise in
two ways. Firstly using your muscles to bring
the arm down, and secondly let the arm drop,
so you are using the weight of the arm, the
force of gravity, to move the arm downwards.

Rotate the whole arm inwards and
then outwards from the shoulder.

Fig. 4.18

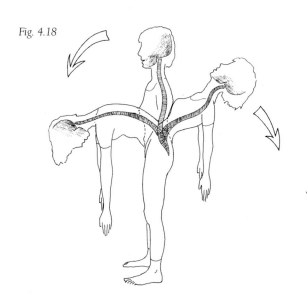

THE SPINE

Bend the spine inwards
and outwards.

Fig.. 4.19

Fig. 4.20

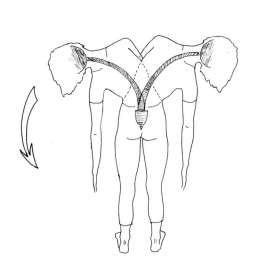

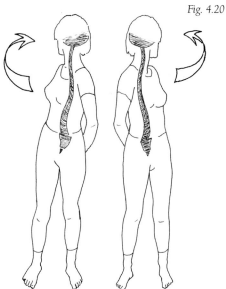

Bend the spine to the left, and
then to the right.

Rotate the head and body round in a clockwise and then in an anti-clockwise direction, so that the spine twists.

• *The Whole Body* •

Prepare to move the body around in different ways, noticing how these different kinds of movements in different combinations make up all our possible movement. Don't stay rigidly with linear movements. When our muscles develop from the embryo they grow in a spiralled way, not in straight lines, and so all our movement patterns tend to have a spirallic quality rather than a linear one. It can be very restricting to think of movement in two dimensional terms, and leads to the militaristic movements of army training. It is more natural to move in a spirallic way and each of our spirallic movements still has an oppositional movement to balance it. The muscles are very adaptable and can move in extremely complex combinations, of which we are quite unaware. We think of some action and as if by magic the muscles combine to perform it more or less perfectly.

Move very slowly and try to be aware of all the different muscles that are coming into play as you move. Visualize the action of the muscle fibres as you move, shortening and lengthening, as the nerve fibres stimulate them. Create a picture of the meat of the muscles, elastic and powerful, contained and protected by the outer sack of the muscle. Feel the stretch on this sack, as you move into positions which are not habitual to you, so they are giving the outer sack of the muscle a gentle stretch. Be aware that for each muscle that is being passively stretched or lengthened in this way there will be opposing muscles shortening. Notice how gravity affects your movements, and how some movements occur just because of the weight of different parts of your body.

Do one movement, and then slowly return to a central, balanced standing position. Then explore another movement, and return to centre. Notice that each action has its balancing action. A movement outwards is balanced by a movement inwards, a twist in one direction is balanced by a twist in another direction. See how many different pairs of actions you can discover, doing each one very slowly, trying to be aware of the muscles involved. You may notice that some actions are easier to perform than the antagonistic actions, so you are bringing into your awareness certain imbalances. These may be particular to you (for instance you may find it easier to bend to the left than to the right), or it may be a more general imbalance, (for example bending the spine inwards tends to happen more easily than bending it outwards). Move all of your body, exploring all possible movements of the legs and arms, the head and neck, and the trunk of the body.

Anti-Gravity Mechanisms

Our muscles are organized so that they balance each other, and they are also organized to bring the body into balance with the force of gravity. We tend to think of gravity as a downward force, which collapses and depresses us, but the reverse is the case. There are reflexes and mechanisms in the structure of the body, which utilize the downward force of gravity to lengthen and strengthen the body in an upward direction. Astronauts have shown us that when they are in space they are unable to stretch and lengthen their bodies. They float around in a semi-foetal position. Without gravity the anti-gravity reflexes in their bodies cannot work.

The most important of these mechanisms occur in the muscles which connect the vertebrae of the neck to the head. The primary function of these muscles is to keep the head balanced on the spine, because the natural tendency of the head is to fall forwards due to the force of gravity acting through it. If you relax all the muscles at the back of the neck the head drops downwards towards the chest, which creates a stretch and lengthening in the muscles in the back of the neck, (*Fig. 4.21*).

It is possible to create a situation where the head is balancing on the neck, causing a very subtle delicate stretching to those muscles at the back of the neck. In this situation the weight of the head is balanced by minute fluctuations in the muscles of the neck, so every delicate adjustment of the head on the spine is creating a subtle massage to the muscles of the neck and back.

So we can use gravity to improve the tone and flexibility of these muscles. These delicate releases set off other anti-gravity reflexes throughout the body; and these mechanisms are fundamental to the proper balance of the body. In most people the mechanisms are badly interfered with, and possibly the most important part of the learning process in the Alexander technique is learning how to restore these delicate mechanisms to good functioning. I shall explain more about this in the chapter entitled 'The Primary Freedom'.

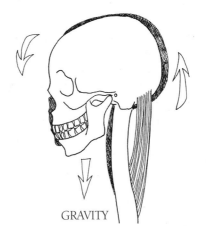

Fig. 4.21

GRAVITY

When Neck Muscles release,
the Head Falls Forwards

We are looking in the musculature of the body for a quality of antagonistic flow, which can be felt in a balanced musculature as a liveliness of the tissues as each of the sets of muscles balance each other through large and minute adjustments. In the preceding exercise you have been putting your body through large movements which cause a lot of lengthening in one set of muscles and shortening in the other set of muscles. But even now, when you are fairly still, reading this book, the muscles are in a state of play maintaining an overall balance. Each movement of your head requires minute adjustments in the muscles of the neck and trunk. When the muscles are in

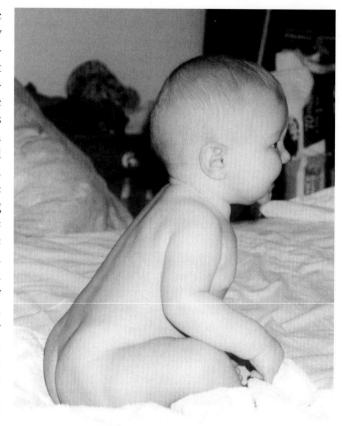

The baby's head is delicately balanced

balance, and there is a good antagonistic flow between opposing sets of muscles throughout the body, then there is a state of good muscle tone in the body. This is experienced in the body as a feeling of wellbeing, internal balance and liveliness.

Imbalance in the Muscles

Imbalance occurs in different ways. Sometimes one set of muscles becomes habitually shortened and the opposing set of muscles may then tend to be collapsed.

Alternatively there may be too much tension and contraction in all the muscles, a general tightening, which results in the outer sacks of the muscles tightening and movement becoming increasingly restricted. Whenever the meat of the muscle is habitually shortened the problem does not lie in the muscle fibre but in the nervous system. For some reason we are sending out impulses for muscle shortening way beyond what is necessary. Our finger is constantly on the doorbell, and to change this we must look to the other end of this chain reaction. We must tackle the problem in the mind, not in the body. Or, more accurately, we must look at how our mental states are creating the physical problems, because it becomes clear from the experiments Alexander made, and from the way in which the muscles and nervous system are a unity, that it is impossible to separate the mind and the body. They are two sides of the same coin, or the same psychophysical unity, as Alexander expressed it.

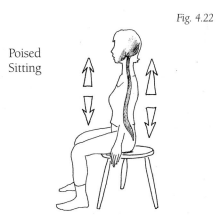

Fig. 4.22

Poised Sitting

When a person is sitting without the back supported, or standing in a balanced way, a slight movement of the head would require minute adjustments in the muscles of the neck and trunk to keep the body stable. If the muscles are in balance back and front then these slight adjustments are like a gentle exercise which keeps the muscles active and in tone, (*Fig. 4.22*) but if the muscles are out of balance it can be very tiring indeed.

When a person slumps in sitting she cannot operate at this refined level, and to maintain this position the muscles which attach the pelvis to the ribs and collar bone are forced to contract while the muscles of the lower back become collapsed or over-extended. This causes weak backs and rounded shoulders if it becomes habitual. The front part of the body becomes pulled down, while the back part becomes collapsed. (*Fig. 4.23a & b*)

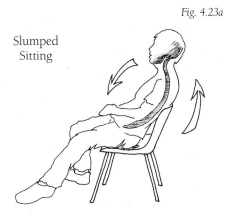

Fig. 4.23a

Slumped Sitting

If this slumping is habitual in a person then, in time, even when she wants to lengthen and release the abdominal muscles, she will be unable to do so, because the meat of the muscle is used to being constantly contracted, and the outer sack of the muscle has contracted also to adapt to the shortened conditions of the meat.

The reverse situation occurs when a person is trying very hard to 'sit up straight'. In this situation the imbalance occurs because the muscles of the back are being unduly contracted, and there is too much tension throughout the whole body. (Fig. 4.24)

Fig. 4.23b   *Fig. 4.24*

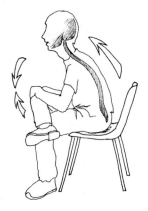
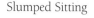

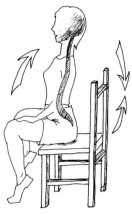

Slumped Sitting   Fixed 'sitting up straight'

THE KINAESTHETIC SENSE

So far we have looked at the process of creating movement in the body, the system of muscle fibres and motor neurons. This system explains how movement occurs. To complete the picture we need to know how the brain and nervous system are informed of this movement, how we have a kinaesthetic sense. In addition to the stimulus and inhibition of movement that occurs via the motor neurons, there is a feedback system, so that the brain and nervous system are constantly informed of the activity of the body, and can adjust the stimulus/inhibitory mechanisms accordingly. Just as there are nerve endings in every muscle fibre which receive stimuli from the nervous system, so there are also nerve endings which send sensory information to the central nervous system. These are called sensory neurons. They are located in the joints, muscles, and tendons and they respond to any movement, stretch or contraction by sending that information to the sensory nerve cells situated in the spinal cord. From there the information is transmitted to the brain. The mechanism by which these sensory neurons work is quite complicated and it is sufficient here to understand the basic principle. (*Fig. 4.25*)

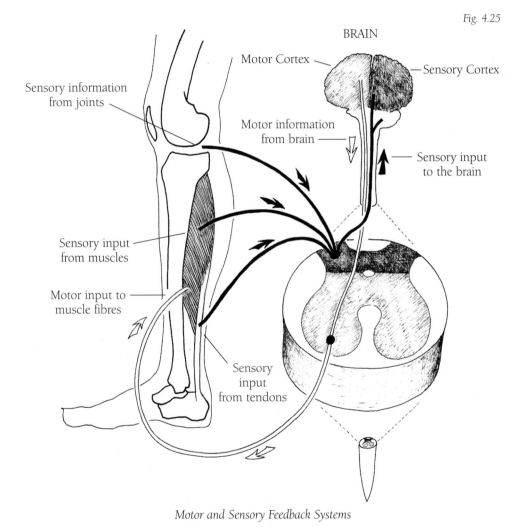

Fig. 4.25

BRAIN

Motor Cortex

Sensory Cortex

Sensory information from joints

Motor information from brain

Sensory input to the brain

Sensory input from muscles

Motor input to muscle fibres

Sensory input from tendons

Motor and Sensory Feedback Systems

A joint is any point at which two bones meet. Highly jointed structures in the body include the neck, wrists and ankles. There are many joints between each delicate vertebra of the neck. The more joints there are, the more sensory information is potentially available. In particular, the neck is highly sensitively tuned in to any movement in the rest of the body, unless the muscles of the neck are too tight, and the joints have become fixed and unable to respond at a sensitive, delicate level to movements of the head and body. When the neck is fixed the amount of sensory information we can receive is reduced.

The sensory neurons in the joints, tendons and muscles form the basis of our kinaesthetic sense. In addition we have a balance mechanism, situated in the inner ear, which is an important part of this kinaesthetic awareness.

Unreliable Sensory Appreciation

But what of the monotony within the human creature's psychophysical self, a monotony caused by the gradual cessation of those sensations concerned with new experiences which have accompanied growth and mobility within the organism since birth? This is, indeed, monotony in its most harmful form, for it goes hand in hand with an increasing degree of stagnation throughout the whole psycho-physical organism. (FMA, CCC)

I hope that you may now have a clearer picture of how the muscles of the body, and the kinaesthetic sense operate. If so, it may be easier to understand why this sense can be so unreliable and faulty. When muscles start to become shortened, the information will be relayed to the brain via the sensory neurons. But when this becomes an habitually fixed state there is no new information for the brain to receive and register. So the sensory mechanism goes to sleep because it has no work to do. The brain is concerned with changes in the muscles, joints and tendons, and so it experiences the chronically shortened state as 'normal' and unchanging. A similar situation arises with the joints; if bones are locked together in a fixed, imbalanced state with no movement, then the brain will register this as the 'normal' state. Only when there is movement and change will the neurological pathways become alive and transmit new information to the brain.

It is common for an Alexander student to complain of how strange it feels when shortened muscles are beginning to release. Subjectively she may experience this as tension or stretch or some other new sensation in the muscle. Objectively, what has happened is that the changes in the muscle as a result of Alexander work have caused new sensory feedback to the brain. The sensory mechanisms of that muscle have begun to wake up and at first it may feel very strange. She is now experiencing the muscle whereas previously she did not experience it at all, although in fact it was then very tense and shortened. Alexander work can result in floods of new sensory information which may be delightful, or which may be so strange that it is difficult for the student to assimilate it all, especially as to begin with that information is not reliable.

To take an example which I mentioned in an earlier chapter, if the bones of the neck are jointed and the muscles contracted so as to make the neck habitually lean slightly to the right, the brain will accommodate to that imbalance and so that position will 'feel right'. When that is released, the information to the brain will be about a movement of the neck to the left. This need not mean that the neck is now leaning to the left. It will just feel that way because it has come out of a rightwards fix, and the muscles around the neck will probably feel strange because they are just beginning to release.

As a student does more work with the Alexander technique, there become less and less fixes and chronic shortenings of muscle. The muscles operate more freely, in a balanced way, and the joints have more mobility and are less likely to be fixed in imbalances, so the information of the sensory neurons is more rich and alive, and it gradually becomes more and more reliable, until what feels right is right. This gradual process of change is the only way a really sound sensory system can be redeveloped.

When the sensory mechanism becomes more refined a person experiences herself in quite a different way. There is an awareness of being more in touch with one's body, and more alive in oneself. There is an increased sensitivity, so if the person is doing something that is putting a strain on the body she will feel this early on in the process and be able to change the situation before it develops into a serious problem. For example, if she slumped, she would feel wrong in this position before very long. The abdomen would feel scrunched up and uncomfortable, and the back would feel pulled.

Many people become students of the Alexander Technique because they suffer from back pain. If the cause of the pain is misuse, then in time it will go away, as they learn an improved use of the self. However, if they misuse themselves again, maybe as a result of some activity that puts a strain on the back if not done carefully, like digging the garden, they will usually get early warning signals from the back, because the sensory mechanism is becoming more reliable. They will feel that it is finding the activity a strain, and they will know they need to take extra care of their use or possibly not continue in the activity that is creating the problem. As the sensory apparatus improves and they become more self-aware, these early warning signals are not ignored, and much pain is avoided.

Mind-Body Unity

It should be clear from the preceding anatomical explanation of the neuromuscular system that it is impossible to talk about the muscles without talking about the nervous system. The motor unit, comprising motor neuron and muscle fibre, operates as a whole, with neurological and physiological aspects; so does the sensory unit comprising muscle fibre and sensory neuron. They are inseparable parts of a whole, and they provide the basis for an understanding that we cannot separate the mind and the body in the way we have tried to do for thousands of years. Our entire culture, our language, our habits of perception are influenced by the assumptions which date back to Plato and beyond, that mind and body can be treated as separate entities. Today, in many different areas of thought, from theoretical physics to psychoanalysis, people are recognising that these assumptions are no longer workable and we must develop a more wholistic understanding of ourselves and the universe. Alexander was one of the first to recognise this internal contradiction which permeates our society and to work with the concept he called 'psychophysical unity', the absolutely inseparable nature of mind and body.

I am not suggesting that the nervous system is the exact equivalent of the mind, but I am saying that our thoughts affect our muscles, and our muscles affect our thoughts in very deep and powerful ways. Practically, this means that when you think that you feel tense, your muscles will respond by contracting even more, whereas if you visualize the muscles in your shoulders releasing they will respond to that mental stimulus by becoming less contracted and tense. It also means that when the muscles in your body release, possibly in the course of an Alexander lesson, there will be an equivalent 'release' in your mental state. One of the commonest pieces of feedback from students is that they feel mentally and emotionally calmer, and this is in direct relation to the level of muscle tension in their bodies.

It is quite easy to see how unified mind and body are when looking at extreme examples. A person who worries a lot and is mentally and emotionally overactive tends to have a lot of muscle tension in the body, whereas the very depressed, exhausted person tends to have a lot of muscle collapse in the body. In between these two extremes there is a kaleidoscope of fascinating variations, but the theme is the same. Our body can be seen as the manifestation of our psyche, and our psyche can be seen as the manifestation of our body. They are both expressions of the self, the whole person.

When the unity of mind and body are accepted it follows that we have to take responsibility for what we are thinking, for how we are using our minds as well as our bodies, because our thoughts are affecting our bodies constantly, and vice versa. There has been a lot of research into this subject in recent years. It has ranged from health studies, where diseases such as cancer are linked to certain mental and emotional attitudes, to sports studies, where athletes have discovered they could improve their performance just as well by visualizing themselves improving, as by physically practising to improve .* This means that we can keep the musculature of our bodies healthy by thinking about healthy movement; and learning to do this is a part of learning the Alexander technique. The quality of our mental attention can help or hinder every activity of our lives, and so it affects the quality of life itself quite fundamentally.

• *Working With Our Thoughts to Release the Muscles* •

Lie down in the semi-supine position as described in Chapter Two. If you have been lying down in semi-supine regularly you will have begun to gather quite a lot of information about yourself. We can now develop this so that we use our minds to create constructive changes in our bodies, to assist the good effect of lying in this position.

Spend the first few minutes, or as long as you feel necessary, getting into a calm listening state, observing yourself as you move into stillness. You may wish to do a body scan, or give attention to the floor contact against your back. Give yourself time to move into that receptive state in which the mind is listening and observing. This will bring about releases throughout the body which you can watch.

Imagine your body is like a lake when it is raining, and all the drops of rain are your thoughts which are disturbing the surface of the lake. Imagine the rain slowly stopping and the raindrops decreasing as your mind stills and the thoughts become less hectic. Eventually, a single drop of rain will send out waves all around it as it lands on the water. When your mind is still, a single thought can affect your body in this clear and powerful way.

When a part of your mind is still and observing what is going on, then you can use another part of your mind to think about your body and encourage releases to occur. You can do this in two ways, by silently talking to yourself, and by visualizing the releases taking place. If you find it difficult to visualize, then work with the verbal suggestions more than the imagistic ones.

*This would not work if the athletes never exercised physically, as the outer sack of the muscle would not be stretched through physical movement and so it would tend to tighten up around the inner meat of the muscle. The thinking process affects the meat of the muscle, as explained above.

Begin with the head and neck. Tell yourself that all the muscles which attach to your skull are in a released and balanced state. Work your way around the head and face, telling yourself how soft and relaxed it is becoming. Here are some suggestions:

My jaw is loose and released.

My ears are relaxed, and so is the area of my head all around them.

My eyes are relaxed, deep inside and on the surface; and the eyelids are relaxing.

My cheeks, nose, eyebrows, forehead, all around the crown of the head, the back of the head, are all becoming soft and relaxed.

Visualize all these changes occurring as you tell yourself about them. Move inside the mouth and think of releases occurring in the tongue and the roof of the mouth and then down into the throat and neck.

Visualize the bones of the neck and all the muscles which attach to the neck and to the head becoming more relaxed and lengthening slightly. Tell yourself how relaxed your neck is. Imagine the back of the neck being very soft and flexible, and how it is being gently stretched and lengthened by the position of your head on the books.

Tell yourself the whole spine is releasing and lengthening. Visualize the curves of the spine releasing from their over-compressed state when you were standing or sitting, and the discs between each vertebra soaking up the body fluid and becoming larger and spongier. The discs make up 25% of the length of the spine, so as they expand the spine lengthens. All the muscles which attach to the spine are lengthening and releasing too. Think of your abdomen becoming soft and relaxed, the whole trunk of your body responding to your positive attention.

Imagine and tell yourself how your back is expanding in all directions, spreading out over the floor, and your chest is releasing and opening out as the back widens. Imagine the muscles themselves, and see the inner meat of the muscle being released and enlivened by the mental attention you are giving it.

Give your attention to your shoulders. Visualize all the muscles between your neck and your shoulders releasing and lengthening, allowing the shoulders to expand outwards. Be careful not to do anything. This is a mental exercise. Think of the muscles under your armpits releasing, so the upper part of the arms are widening away from the rib-cage, allowing more movement of the ribs and freedom in the breathing. Visualize the shoulder socket, where the upper arm attaches, being free and released so that this allows the widening process to develop even more. Tell yourself that the muscles of the arms and hands are releasing, visualizing releases in the muscles and in the elbow, wrist and finger joints.

Now give your attention to your legs and pelvis. Think of the pelvic girdle of the body being free and released and all the muscles around the hip joint releasing. See the leg as two upright sides of a triangle with the base of the triangle on the floor, so the feet and the back are supporting the sides of the triangle, (Fig. 4.26).

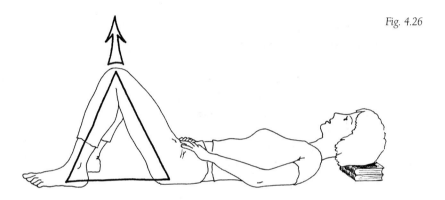

Fig. 4.26

See the leg as two upright sides of a triangle with the base of the triangle on the floor. Send the knees up towards the ceiling.

Imagine these two sides, your upper and lower leg, getting longer as the muscles and joints release and visualize the knees moving up towards the ceiling above you as this releasing process occurs. Imagine there are strings attached to your knees, gently pulling your legs upwards, allowing lengthening and release in hips, ankles and muscles of the legs.

Work out some more releasing ideas of your own that you can play with. All the time you are working with these ideas, keep that observant part of your mind watching the changes that occur as you give your body this positive attention.

When you get up from semi-supine notice the differences in your mind and body as you gently begin to move again. Record any interesting discoveries or changes that occurred in your notebook.

• *Working with our Thoughts to Enliven the Muscles* •

In the last exercise your attention was on releasing and lengthening contracted muscles and joints, and the Alexander technique does emphasize working with release in this way. However it is possible to work with your mind on your muscles in very different ways, ways which athletes are discovering to be very effective. To experience the contrast you may occasionally like to experiment with thinking in quite a different way. After you have been lying in semi-supine for a while, observing yourself and working with releasing ideas, change your thinking process as follows.

Imagine you are going for a lovely walk on a sunny day in the countryside. Visualize your legs moving along the path, your arms swinging by your sides. Enjoy the feeling of movement in your body. Because you are enjoying swinging your arms so much let them swing right round in circles for a while. Feel the pleasant circular movement on the shoulder joints gently stretching the chest muscles as each arm goes backwards. Decide you would like to run and move smoothly into running, visualizing your body flowing smoothly and freely. Enjoy all the physical sensations you associate with running lightly in this way. Now you are getting quite hot and fortunately there is a very safe lake or river close by, which is just the right temperature to encourage you in for a swim. Now visualize and experience your body swimming through the water, the movements of your arms and legs and your whole body moving easily through the liquid surrounding you. Swim on your back and on your front, experiencing as many different strokes as you can. When you get out a towel miraculously appears for you to dry yourself on, and because you are feeling so good you do a little dance to express your pleasure.

You may feel quite exhausted after this exercise! People who don't exercise much and tend to be lethargic will benefit more from this visualization than people who enjoy regular exercise. If you do feel exhausted it may be easier for you to take one activity at a time and experience the effect of visualizing it upon your body. For people who tend to be overactive and tense it is more useful to visualize the releases in the muscles and joints when you are lying in semi-supine, and in general this is the emphasis we work with in the technique.

Chapter Five

Alexander's Experiments

In this chapter I am going, in as simple a way as I can, to go through some of Alexander's practical experiments which led him to the discoveries about good use and mis-use that are the foundation of his technique.

Alexander used three mirrors to help him make his observations, one to give him a front view and two to give him side views. If you can arrange two full length mirrors so that you have a good profile view of yourself in addition to a front view this will work very well. Otherwise one full length mirror plus a hand mirror will do. If you do not have a full length mirror you can work with a half mirror, as most of your attention will be on your head and neck.

• *Your Use With Your Voice* •

Stand in front of the mirror with your eyes closed. Get a sensory picture of how you appear, the position of your feet, whether your shoulders are level or not, whether your head is straight or tilted. Now open your eyes and check how accurate your kinaesthetic information is.

It is important that you observe yourself in as much detail as possible. Stand with your feet hip width apart, facing the mirror. Start talking into the mirror as though you were addressing a friend. Tell your image what you plan to do today, or tomorrow, or what you had for breakfast, or what you like to cook for your favourite meal. Talk about something that is not too intellectually demanding! The important thing is that you are able to observe yourself at the same time as talking, so you cannot read from a script. Later you could try talking about something that is more demanding and notice if that creates differences in your muscle patterns.

Observe what is happening in your face, neck and shoulders when you talk. Notice the movements of the jaw and whether you can see other muscles of the face working. Notice any movement of the head as you speak, and any movement of the shoulders. Do you feel tense anywhere when you talk? Talk for a sentence or two and observe, and then be silent and observe, noticing the difference, visually and kinaesthetically, between the two states.

Repeat all this using a side view. Notice any movement of the head. Look also at the jaw from the side and the arrangement in profile of the jaw and neck. See which muscles tense when you speak, and see whether this tension is appropriate or whether you think some muscles seem too tense. A lot of people habitually hold their jaws very very tight and this becomes more noticeable when talking, and then when stopping talking. (This is a very good exercise to do in pairs, if possible, with another person observing you in addition to yourself. It is then possible to compare the differences in tension that different people exhibit when talking.)

Now repeat all these experiments from the front and the side, but speaking in a very loud voice, as though you were on stage, addressing hundreds of people. Note the differences between speaking quietly and speaking loudly.

Alexander noticed that when he did similar experiments he pulled his head back and down when he spoke loudly. He then noticed that he also pulled his head back and down when he spoke normally, but this was a subtler, less noticeable movement of which he was not aware until after he had observed it when he spoke loudly. In addition to pulling his head back he sucked in the air to breathe, and the pulling of his head backwards caused the larynx (throat area) to be depressed.

Now repeat the exercises looking for the tendency to pull the head back and down before speaking loudly, and any other observations as well. A good way to notice head movement is to watch the hair as it falls on the neck. Any movement of the hair must involve a movement of the head. You will probably find that you too manifest this habitual tendency to pull the head back and down. Another way of observing what happens to your head and neck when speaking loudly is to place one hand on the back of the neck, resting it gently against the neck and the back of the head, and then shout out your name. Feel with your hand what goes on in the muscles at the back of the neck and head when you shout. You will probably feel a tightening of the muscles in the neck. When you are aware of your habitual use when shouting or speaking loudly, see whether you can observe a subtler version of the same use when you are speaking normally.

Having observed the relationship of the head and neck when speaking, go on to look at what happens to the rest of your body. Notice what happens to your shoulders and arms, your chest, your back, your stomach, your legs and feet. First speak quietly, and then speak as loudly as you can.

When Alexander did these experiments he noticed that he raised his chest, and arched and narrowed his back, (*Fig. 5.1*). These misuses were pronounced when he was speaking loudly and they were still there to a lesser extent when speaking normally. He also used his legs, feet and toes in ways that involved undue muscle tension, and interfered with his balance. Raising the chest and narrowing the back were a part of the total pattern of pulling the head back and gasping for breath. These are very common tendencies and it is likely you will find you do the same. However we don't all misuse our bodies in precisely the same way. For example, some people tend to hold their shoulders back, while others pull them forwards. Although the tendency to pull the head back is almost universal, the total pattern of misuse differs for each individual. Spend a little time exploring your own habits, and make notes of what they are.

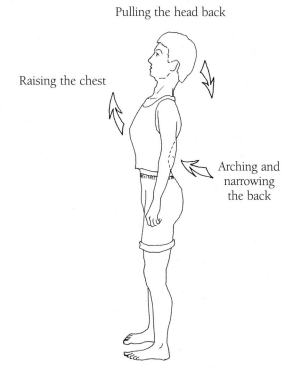

Fig. 5.1

Pulling the head back

Raising the chest

Arching and narrowing the back

When Alexander was making these discoveries about himself he thought they were his individual problems, and that most other people did not have these faults. Later, when he began teaching his method to other people, he realized that virtually everyone tends to pull the head back whenever they have to carry out even a relatively simple activity, and that pulling the head back was the major misuse that occurred in all people. He learnt this through the long experience of working on himself and on others. Pulling the head back is the primary misuse from which all the other misuses followed, and so if this primary misuse could be stopped, the other secondary misuses might also be prevented.

• Unreliable Sensory Appreciation •

As you might expect, the next part of Alexander's research involved trying to speak without pulling the head back. This proved to be easier said than done.

See if you can speak loudly without pulling your head back. First of all try doing this without the help of the mirror, just using your own kinaesthetic awareness. When you think you have succeeded in not pulling your head back - when it 'feels' right - look in the mirror and see whether you really have succeeded or not.

After you have used your visual sense, experience what the back of the head and neck feel like to touch, by resting your hand gently against them; now speak loudly.

At this point Alexander discovered what we discussed at length in the last chapter, that he couldn't rely on his feelings. Even when he thought he had got it right, careful observation proved that he was still pulling his head back. He began to be aware of the power of habit, and the lack of conscious control we have over our movements when they are operating against an habitual movement. This was an enormous discovery. Its implications, and how Alexander solved this dilemma, shall be dealt with in following chapters.

• Sitting and Standing •

If you have had any individual work from an Alexander teacher it is more than likely that you have done some work with the simple movements of sitting down in a chair and standing up again. The reason teachers like to use these movements a lot in their work is because sitting down and standing up are simple everyday activities in which, nevertheless, we tend to misuse ourselves very badly. They can therefore help a student to change by working with these movements.

Place a chair in front of the mirror. Stand in front of the chair so that you are able to sit down on the chair without moving your feet. Observe yourself in standing and then sit down. At first notice the position of the head relative to the body. To judge whether you have pulled your head back from this position, notice whether you see more of the front of your neck, and whether your chin tilts upwards a little. This means you are tilting the head backwards. Stand up again and notice the head and neck once more. Also notice what you are doing with your bottom, with your legs, especially the knees, and with your arms, shoulders, chest and the trunk of the body. Make detailed observations in a similar way to the work you did in the previous exercise.

Now make your observations of yourself in profile. Once again, movement of the hair is the best indication of movement of the head. If the hair moves down the neck or back as you sit and stand, then you are pulling your head back. In this position it is easier to see what is happening to your spine as you sit down. Does it bend and in what way? Build up a picture of your use in this movement.

Again, see whether you can manage to sit down without pulling the head back. First of all do it without using the mirror. See if it feels that the head is not pulled back and down. When it feels right, test this by using the mirror to monitor your observations. If it looks as though you are not pulling the head back, place your hand on the back of your neck and head as you sit, and feel whether the muscles are tightening at the back of your neck when you sit down. (*Fig. 5.2*)

Fig. 5.2

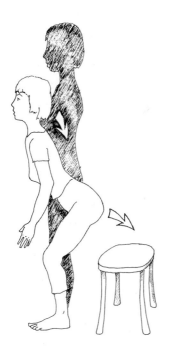
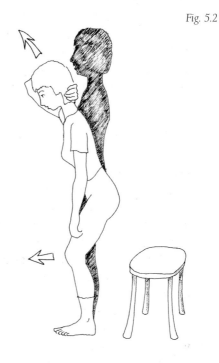

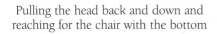
Pulling the head back and down and reaching for the chair with the bottom

Sending the head forwards an up, whilst bending at the hips, knees and ankles

In addition to the observations you are making about your physical use, notice the effect upon you mentally of observing yourself. Do you find working with a mirror is difficult? Are you concerned that you want to get it 'right' or are you simply curious about how you are using yourself. Notice your mental attitudes to carrying out these experiments.

The quality of observation required for these experiments is very subtle and refined. Most people pull their heads back, but it is hardly noticeable. If you find you cannot see these misuses, I suggest you work with another person or, preferably, you ask an Alexander teacher to point them out to you. Sometimes a student tries to stop pulling the head back by fixing the neck quite rigidly. This creates a lot of unhelpful muscular tension, and is another way of shortening and tightening the muscles at the back of the neck, which is in effect the same as pulling the head back. When you place your hand on the back of the head and neck you may be able to feel this tightening of the musculature.

Although there has been a certain element of 'trying to get it right' in these experiments, they are best seen as useful observations, so that you do not bring all the tension into your activity that 'trying to get it right' implies. We are primarily concerned with what is going wrong, rather than with trying to get it right. Until we are clear about what goes wrong we cannot work out a means to change this wrong use. The reason I have suggested you try to get it right is precisely because such an effort is more or less doomed. Alexander tried to get it right and realised the futility of this approach, because habitual use influenced his behaviour much more powerfully than his attempt to get right something that was contrary to the force of habit. Indeed his attempt to get it right only brought a further level of tension into the activity. You may have observed this for yourself.

ALEXANDER'S SOLUTIONS

People don't do what they feel to be wrong when they are trying to be right. (FMA, UCL)

From Feeling to Thinking

The work Alexander did with mirrors, and later when he worked with other people, enabled him to discover a series of related wrongs or misuses that human beings, or certainly the civilized Western ones, tend to employ. The primary and universal misuse is the tendency to pull the head back and down, causing the back to shorten and narrow. Everyone has individual variations, but this was the major 'doing' that he found was going wrong, the habitual misuse that would occur in response to a stimulus, such as the stimulus to speak loudly, or to sit down in a chair, or the stimulus of a loud noise, such as the doorbell ringing, in fact, quite simply, the stimulus to react in any way at all. In all of his pupils he found it had become a fixed pattern of misuse. If this tightening and dis-coördinating pattern could be replaced by a relationship of the head, neck and back which allowed the spine to lengthen and the back to widen, then this would bring about an overall improvement in the use of the self which would result in an improvement in overall functioning.

Alexander spent many painstaking years working on himself to find out what he was doing that was causing his functional problems. He emphasized that the only way we can make changes is to get to know what is going wrong. He discovered that not only was he using himself wrongly, but also that the sensory information by means of which he had hoped to correct the wrong use was in itself faulty, and so he could not rely on it to make the changes he desired. He spent a lot of time practising doing the activity in what he thought was the right way, only to discover over and over again that his habitual misuse got the better of him. As soon as he thought about doing the activity of reciting, his nervous system geared itself up to its old habitual response, and his attempt at a new response fell by the wayside. It was as a result of his repeated failures that he began to understand the nature of faulty sensory appreciation, because even though he felt he was doing it right, careful observation in the mirror proved that he was still doing it wrong.

He had to find some other way to bring about a change in his use, and this led him to the next major discovery around which his technique evolved.

Means and Ends

Eventually he decided that instead of trying to do it right, he should give all his attention to stopping doing it wrong. So instead of trying to recite without pulling his head back, he gave all his attention to not pulling his head back, and didn't even attempt to recite. This subtle change of approach is central to his technique. It emphasizes the process of changing rather than the results. Alexander called this paying attention to the 'means whereby', rather than 'endgaining'.

In addition he realized that he had to find a way of changing that did not rely upon his sensory mechanism, and so instead of trying to do the right thing he experimented with thinking the right thing, and doing nothing. It was by working in this way that he recognized the inseparable nature of mind and body, or in his words a 'psychophysical unity'. By thinking the appropriate thoughts, changes would occur in the musculature. Biofeedback machines which can register the level of muscular tension in the body have since demonstrated precisely these discoveries, which Alexander made through developing his own self-awareness.

In his initial experiments Alexander had tried to stop pulling the head back and down, by putting it forwards and up. This hadn't worked. Now he simply thought that he wanted his head to go forwards and up, and he did not want it to go back and down, and he did nothing at all except check in the mirror to see whether this was preventing the wrong use. He described this as giving 'Directions' to his nervous system. Whenever he thought about reciting he simply decided not to, so as not to stimulate the old wrong use, and he called this 'Inhibition'. He continued for a long time with this process of saying 'No' whenever the old stimulus to recite occurred, at the same time thinking the thoughts that would prevent the old misuses from being triggered into action. By these means, and very gradually, the old habitual reaction to the stimulus to recite became less powerful and dominant, and he could maintain the improved use for longer periods. Eventually he could inhibit the old misuses successfully enough to do something, such as sit down, recite, or remain standing while maintaining the new improved use, the important emphasis being upon how he did the activity, not upon the end of having accomplished the activity.

The painstaking attention to the subtleties of his mind and body, and the patience with which Alexander approached this problem is quite awe inspiring. By doing nothing, refusing to react to an habitual stimulus, and thinking in ways that would encourage the change in use, Alexander was in effect intervening in the powerful instinctual responses of his nervous system. He did this with very little understanding of anatomy and physiology. He did not know why from a scientific point of view his experiments successfully altered the reactions of his nervous system. Nevertheless he realized through his observations and experiments that he had discovered something very remarkable about the workings of the human organism, and how it was possible to move from an instinctual or habitual response, to one that was under conscious control and direction.

The first book Alexander wrote was called *Man's Supreme Inheritance*. Our inheritance is precisely this ability to move from an instinctual and habitual use of our organism, to one that is guided by conscious awareness. He continued this theme in his second book which is called *Constructive Conscious Control of the Individual*. It is by means of our consciousness that we can genuinely create changes at a very fundamental level, firstly in the way we use the psychophysical organism, and then in any other areas in which we want to function with conscious awareness and choice, not simply from habit.

From Thinking to Feeling

The gap between instinctive and conscious control of the self must be bridged . . . Moreover and all important, the prerequisite to each step in this process is the restoration of trustworthiness to the human sensorium without which a human being could not register experience so as to be able to test its validity. (FMA, *CCC*)

It may appear that by moving from habitual to conscious control Alexander was eliminating the role of sensory feelings altogether. But this was not the case. He saw his work as re-educating the psychophysical mechanism so that the sensations became reliable once more. A developed awareness of his sensory mechanism was absolutely necessary to the process of changing. After all, he could not even know that the information of his senses was unreliable if he didn't get that information, and then monitor it against his visual information.

In the process of changing from the old habitual use to the new improved use, Alexander allowed his body to feel something quite new and unfamiliar. He allowed his body to experience his head being forwards and up and his back lengthening and widening. This is the experience that an Alexander teacher gives to his students. Because it is such an unfamiliar feeling it can feel quite awkward and wrong to begin with, but as the body gets used to the changes the new use will begin to feel more familiar. At this point the sensory information becomes more reliable, because as a good use of the self begins to feel familiar it also begins to feel right. We can trust the information of the senses once again and allow the reasoning and the feeling to work together in harmony.

Chapter Six

The Primary Freedom

This led me to discover that a particular relativity of the head to the neck and the head and neck to other parts of the organism tended to improve general use and functioning of the organism as a whole, and that the motivation for this use was from the head downwards, and, further, that any other particular relativity tended towards the opposite effect.   (FMA, UCL)

Alexander discovered that there is a universal tendency in human beings to pull the head back, so much so, that in many individuals the muscles which pull the head back have become chronically shortened, and unable to release naturally. He then worked out how to stop this habitual misuse. In addition to this primary misuse he detected many other related misuses of the body which tended to vary slightly from individual to individual. But the way the head balances on the neck is the primary mechanism to understand. Although Alexander himself never used anatomical explanations in his work, I think it is a very useful way of understanding this central concept, and we shall explore it anatomically and in other ways in this chapter.

• *Experiencing the Weight of the Head* •

Lie down in the semi-supine position and allow yourself to relax. Be particularly aware of the weight of the head on the books. When you feel sufficiently relaxed lift the head from the books. Do this as slowly as it is possible to do, as though you were very very weak and had only the minimum of strength to perform this manoeuvre. If you do it very slowly indeed, you may be able to feel each individual muscle that comes into play in order to lift the head, and you may be able to feel just what a lot of work is required to lift the head because it is so heavy. Do not repeat this exercise as it causes a lot of unwanted muscular contraction in the front of the neck, which we do not want to encourage.

If you are able to work with another person, take it in turns to lie down while one person lifts the head of the person lying down. When you lift the head, do it very slowly and very gently. If you do it quickly and thoughtlessly, the person who is lying down will be unable to avoid tightening the muscles in the front of the neck and holding the head up himself, so you will not be able to get an accurate sense of the weight of the head.

GRAVITY

Fig. 6.1

FORWARDS AND UP

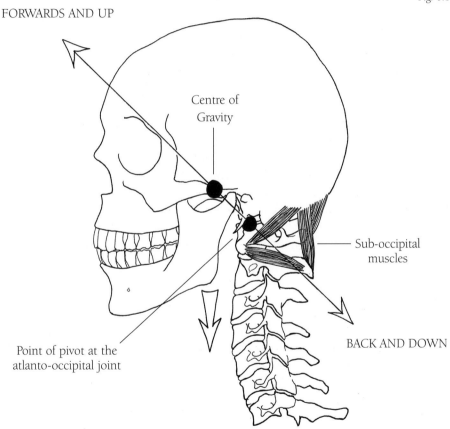

The Anatomical Relationship of the Head to the Neck

The weight of the head is about ten to twelve pounds. It is a very heavy part of us. Next time you go shopping see if you can find a 10 lb bag of potatoes to lift so that you can get some experience of how heavy the head is. The head balances on top of the spine, the point of pivot being called the Atlanto-occipital joint. The way it is organized on the spine is such that the centre of gravity of the head is forward of the point of pivot of the skull on the top vertebrae of the spine. (See *Fig. 6.1*). So the head has a tendency to fall forwards all the time. What stops it doing so are the muscles that connect the back of the skull to other parts of the skeleton. If someone falls asleep in the sitting position the head will fall forwards as these muscles release. We say he has 'nodded off', which is exactly what the head

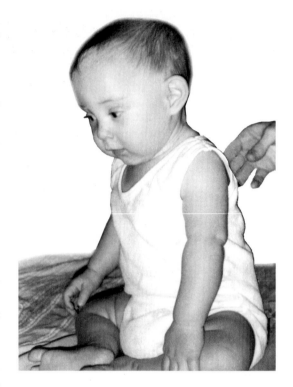

Baby learning to sit by balancing head

does when we fall asleep in this way. When we are awake we are not aware of the muscles that are working to keep the head on, because this activity is so automatic and habitual to the waking state.

The muscles which connect the skull to the rest of the body are in several layers. On the deep inner layer are a group of small delicate muscles, which attach the skull to the first two vertebrae of the spine, and they are called the sub-occipitals. The function of these muscles is to keep the head balanced on the spine in a delicate way. The first vertebra of the spine is jointed to the skull in such a way that the head can gently nod up and down a short distance, and the second vertebra allows the head to rotate a little. To nod the head more, or rotate the head further would require more movement of the other neck vertebrae. When the weight of the head is balanced by the gentle fluctuating activity of the sub-occipital muscles, it encourages a lengthening of all the muscles in the neck and the back. Every time the head rotates slightly forwards there is a gentle stretch on the sub-occipitals, and so on the other muscles of the neck and back. This subtle lengthening of the muscles of the neck and back creates releases throughout the torso, and stimulates other anti-gravity reflexes in the body, freeing the ribs so that the breathing mechanisms are energized, and allowing the possibility of increased release and lengthening throughout the musculature. In this way the force of gravity becomes an aid to the lengthening and strengthening of the musculature of the body.

If you watch very young children when they are learning to sit, and later to stand, and then to walk, you can observe that they have not yet developed the strength in their neck and back muscles in the way adults have. Nor have they developed a habitual tendency to pull the head back. What these children can be seen to be doing is learning to balance the heavy weight of the head on the neck, using the delicate sub-occipital muscles designed for that purpose. Their whole organisms are focused upon learning this new act of balancing. And it is this skill that we have to relearn.

In the layers of muscle above the delicate sub-occipital muscles are much stronger muscles which attach to the lower vertebrae of the spine and to the shoulder blades, and collar bone, (Fig. 6.2). Once we have learnt to walk we start learning to do more demanding actions, like running, carrying heavy objects, sitting down in chairs, and standing up again. All these require great feats of balance for our heads, and they also require the use of more powerful muscles. Whenever one of these demanding actions is necessary we tend to pull the head back, by shortening and tightening these larger more powerful muscles.

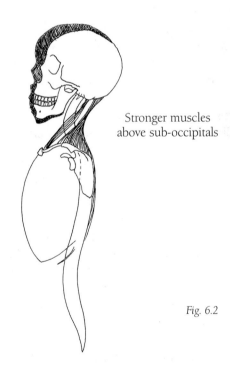

Stronger muscles above sub-occipitals

Fig. 6.2

Stronger muscles contract to pull head back down

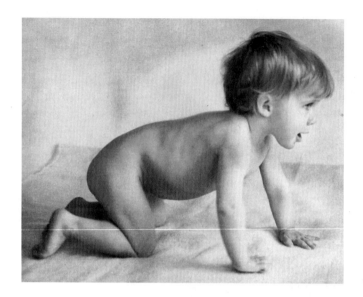

When a child learns
to walk . . .

. . . its whole organism
is focussed . . .

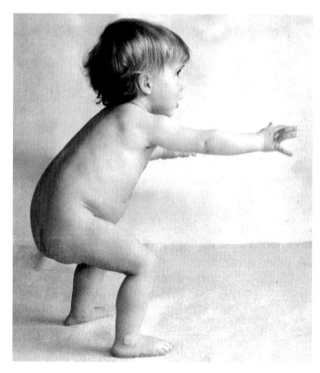

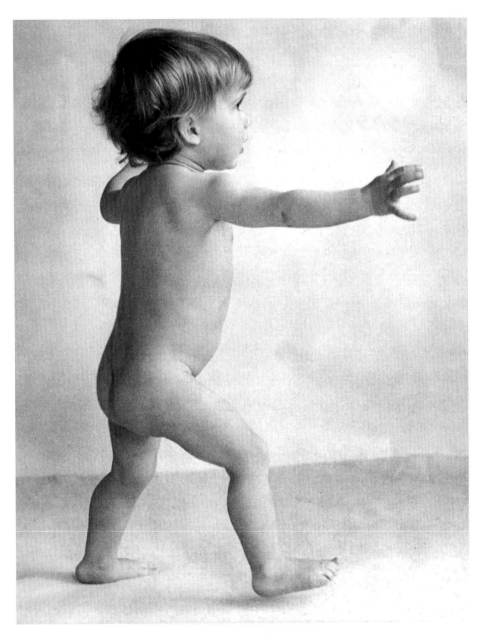

. . . upon balancing the heavy weight of the head on the spine.

• Giving Your Attention to the Weight of the Head •

Find a heavy book and place it on your head, holding it gently with one hand. Stand still and notice the effect on your body of having this weight on your head. Then slowly walk around feeling the balance of the book on the head, and how it affects your use to have this weight to consider in your movement. Experiment with taking your hand away, but notice if you are getting caught up with the idea of 'succeeding'. The important thing to notice is what it feels like to have your attention on balancing a weight on the head. This is the closest we can get to repeating our experience as an infant learning to walk. Notice how every muscle is poised and directed into maintaining the balance. (I am not recommending this as a regular exercise, in the way schools of posture do! I simply want you to experience a little more weight on your head.)

Now imagine that you have some thick straps and you are going to strap this heavy book onto your head by straps that go under the arms, and under the crutch, so it cannot fall off. It is now possible to move without that careful attention, and this is similar to the average person's everyday movements.

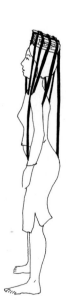

Fig. 6.3

Strapping the head onto the body, by shortening the larger muscles of the neck and back, is analogous to strapping the book onto the head in the above experiment (*Fig. 6.3*). And this is an example of how most people use themselves all the time. The heavy weight of the book represents the heavy weight of the head, something which has become so 'normal' that it is strapped onto the body and no longer taken into account. It may be possible to do things more quickly, with your head strapped on by the larger muscles of the neck and back, but it is not doing you so much good as when

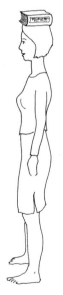

Finely balanced   Unbalanced

you give attention to your balance, and the movements of the body are coordinated and integrated by the attention upon the head. Strapping the head onto the body, causes fixing in the joints of the neck, and in the muscles, all of which reduces the mobility and freedom of the head and neck, which in turn reduces the stimulation of the sensory neurons, and so less information is available to the nervous system about what is going on in the body.

• *The Startle Response* •

Sit in a relaxed and comfortable way. Place your hand gently on the back of your neck. Ask a friend to slam a door or shout loudly without giving you any warning. You may find you pull your head back in anticipation of the unpleasant experience. Or you may be clever enough to inhibit your startle response when the noise occurs. But if you don't think of inhibiting you will find the muscles at the back of your neck tighten.

One of the reflex responses of the body occurs in response to stress or shock. There is a tightening and shortening beginning in the muscles of the head and neck and spreading throughout the body. The head is pulled back and down, the shoulders are raised, the arms stiffen and the knees bend. Whenever we are subjected to minor nervous stress, such as a sudden noise like the slamming of a door, we react reflexly in this way. And of course the greater the stress the more likely this is to happen. So our response to physical and emotional stress is to pull the head back and down. It is as though we wish to pull the heavy head as close as possible to the point of pivot, which makes the head mechanically more stable and 'safer', whenever we are startled, or when we have to do something mechanically demanding of the stability of our structure.

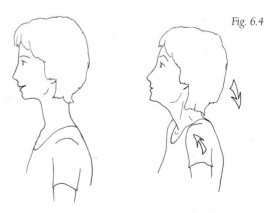

Fig. 6.4

The Startle Reflex

When we pull the head back and down, whether as a result of emotional or physical stress, the spine is compressed because the muscles in the back and front of our bodies tighten. All this creates lack of coordination in the body, and the shortening and narrowing of the back which Alexander described. If we do not release out of this pulled down state, then the muscles involved become habitually contracted.

When the strong powerful muscles in the back of the neck become habitually contracted, the delicate sub-occipital muscles are necessarily also shortened and so they are not able to do their sensitive balancing of the head on the spine even when the body is relatively at rest, sitting or standing. So the head is not only pulled back, it becomes fixed back because the muscles have contracted and not released. It is quite easy to demonstrate the aging process by looking at it from this point of view. (*Fig. 6.5*)

The Aging Process

Fig.6.5

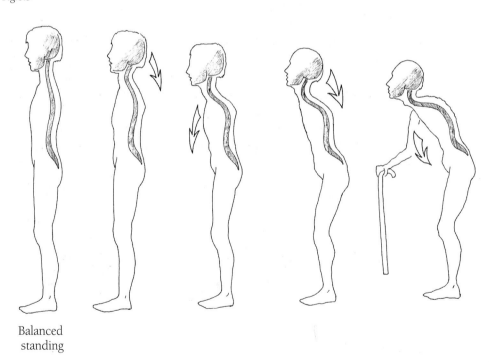

Balanced
standing

Head remains pulled back. Body adjusts by collapsing forward and down.

Primary Control

The employment of the primary control conditions all other reactions, brings the conditioning factor under conscious direction, and enables the individual to take possession of his own potentialities. It converts the fact of conditioned reflexes from a principle of external enslavement into a means of vital freedom.   Prof. J.Dewey (Introduction *UOS*)

To undo these problems, we have to learn to release the powerful muscles in the neck and back, and allow the sub-occipital muscles to do their delicate work of balancing the head on the spine. Lying down in semi-supine is a good way of helping this process. The contact of the back against the floor and the gentle stretch on the neck, because the head is resting on books, encourages release in the muscles of the neck and back. We also need to learn how to operate with the minimum necessary tensions in these muscles when we are upright and in movement. Learning how to do this is learning how to improve the primary control of the use of the self, and it this skill that Alexander teachers are trained to teach.

To counteract the tendency to pull the head back and down, Alexander experimented with putting the head forward. He found this helped, but that if he put it too far forward it would then be going forward and down and causing an equivalent depression in the larynx as if he were to pull the head back. (*Fig. 6.6*). He discovered that there was a particular dynamic arrangement of the head to the neck and back, which freed the whole torso and created a lengthening and widening throughout the back, and that this relationship was primary to all others in the use of the body.

Fig. 6.6

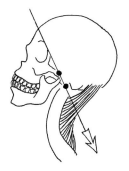
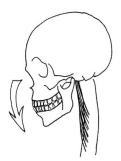
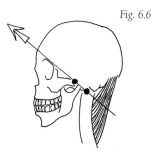

Back and down   Forwards and down   Forwards and up

Three Directions of the Head

He concluded that for the primary control to be working well, the head should be going forwards and up in such a way that the back lengthened and widened.

If you look at the diagram of the head and neck, (*Fig. 6.1*), you can see the mechanics of this discovery. The line connecting the Centre of Gravity of the head to the point of pivot (Atlanto-occipital joint), gives the direction of 'back and down', when we are pulling the head back, or the opposite direction 'forwards and up', when we inhibit that reflex response and direct the Centre of Gravity of the head away from the point of pivot. When the direction of the head is forwards and up, the precisely opposite direction to the head being pulled back and down, there is a situation of mechanical advantage. When the head is directed correctly the muscles of the whole torso receive a lengthening stretch, which allows the spine to be lengthened rather than compressed as it is by the reflex response of pulling the head back. (*Fig. 6.7*)

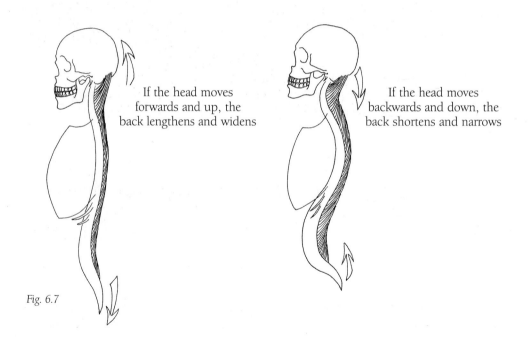

If the head moves forwards and up, the back lengthens and widens

If the head moves backwards and down, the back shortens and narrows

Fig. 6.7

When the head is releasing 'forwards and up', all the releasing mechanisms throughout the body are stimulated, and the body moves as a whole in a coordinated and integrated way, with the head leading the movement. In all vertebrates the head is the primary organiser of movement. This is easy to see in four legged animals. A cat or a dog will follow its nose, eyes, or ears. The head moves as a result of a sensory stimulus, and the body organises itself around the movement of the head, in the horizontal plane. It is easy to see in a four legged animal that the spine is pulled along behind the head. In humans we go forwards in the horizontal plane, and we need also to lengthen the spine upwards in the vertical plane. This is a more complex task, and most adults have lost the ability to perform it well.

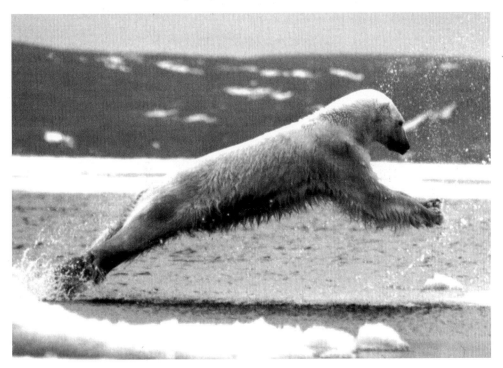

Polar bear leaps 'head first' across the ice

If the primary control is working well in a person, there is an integrating and releasing activity occurring all the time throughout the mind and body, which is usually experienced as a feeling of lengthening and widening in the torso and of 'going up', and this is the essence of good use. Movement becomes more poised, lighter and freer. What stops the primary control working well is that we interfere with its natural functioning. We interfere in the ways explored in the last chapter, by pulling the head back and down, shortening and narrowing the back, or by allowing a reflex response such as the startle pattern to be a 'fixed' state in our bodies. By releasing ourselves from these interferences we discover our natural ability for good use. When the primary control is functioning without interference it gives rise to the greatest ease of movement. The head is freely balanced on the spine, and the mind and body experience a parallel freedom and flexibility. The primary control then gives rise to the primary freedom of the body.

In order to regain this freedom of thought and action we need to go back to the basics of life. We need to learn how to breathe, sit, stand, walk and talk with the same total attention of a baby, and with the conceptual skills of an adult. And so we go through a rebirth, relearning the fundamentals, and unlearning the interferences that we no longer choose to be part of our habitual response pattern.

Leading with the Head

The birth of the human being normally begins with the head pushing its way down the birth canal, followed by the wriggling body. Life begins with movement, firstly as an embryo and then as a newly born baby. At the very beginning of life we experience the primacy of the head, organizing our movement. Once born, the next new activity is breathing air into the lungs, which may be accompanied by the first use of the voice. Moving, breathing and using the voice were all elements of Alexander's teaching. Learning to do these simple and fundamental activities of living with ease and freedom makes the Alexander technique a strong foundation upon which other activities of life can be developed. It is not a foundation in the sense of something heavy and fixed, but in the sense of something absolutely fundamental to every aspect of life, which can then be applied to everything else that we do..

The importance of the head as the organiser of all our movements was discovered by Alexander in his practical work on himself and with pupils, and at the same time it was discovered by G.E. Coghill, a biologist researching into animal organisms, and its application is universal throughout the animal kingdom. If we approach all our movement with the ability to operate the primary control without interference, leading with the head, and lengthening and widening the back, then all our movements can be a source of fulfilment and enrichment.

Opposite: *The meercat needs a good view of potential predators, so the head moves up and the spine lengthens*

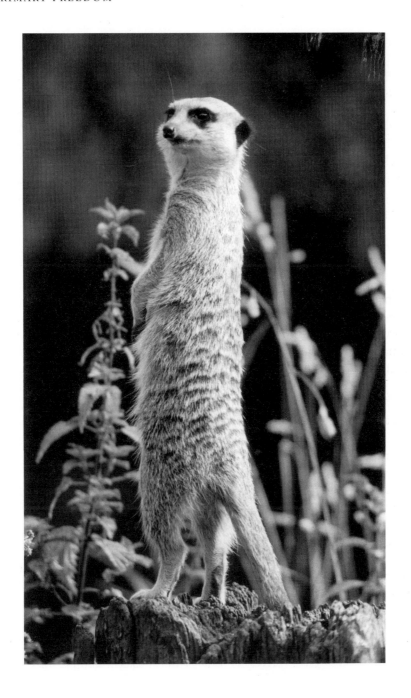

The Breathing Man

As a matter of fact, given the perfect co-ordination of parts as required by my system, breathing is a subordinate operation which will perform itself.. (FMA,MSI)

When Alexander discovered how to get the primary control working well in his organism, and with this learned to release his individual interferences and misuse patterns, he found that his voice and respiratory problems disappeared. He was able to recite for long periods without becoming hoarse, and he no longer sucked the air in through his mouth when he breathed, but breathed through his nose easily. His respiratory capacity increased, and he had plenty of energy and liveliness in his mind and body. When he was getting quite old a young boy who met Alexander, asked his mother, 'Who is that young man, with grey hair?' His movements were free and flexible throughout his life, not the kind of movements associated with old age. Alexander's own experience showed him that he had something very remarkable to offer the human race.

The effect of the spine lengthening is that all the muscles that attach to the spine are given a gentle stretch, and the discs in between the vertebrae of the spine are able to expand and regenerate, encouraging further lengthening, so there is a releasing process that takes place throughout the torso. The increased length of the spine opens out the ribs and this encourages a freer movement of the ribs in breathing. This movement of the ribs creates a gentle massage on all the muscles connected to the ribs, and as these muscles lengthen and release there is a lengthening and widening throughout the torso. The breathing naturally improves under these changed conditions. (*Fig. 6.8*)

When Alexander began teaching his technique to others, he became known as 'The Breathing Man', partly because his own breathing mechanism was so well co-ordinated, and partly because in his early teaching days he focused a lot on re-education of the respiratory mechanism.

There are lots and lots of breathing techniques available today. Some are directed towards actors and singers, and some are more connected with relaxation and 'deep breathing'. Alexander's approach to breathing is consistent with his approach to all activity. If we stop doing the wrong thing, the right thing will do itself. He particularly stressed this in relation to breathing, because good breathing is a secondary effect of operating with good use. Breathing exercises and methods which deal specifically with breathing can interfere with the natural capacity of the organism to 'be breathed'. Breathing should not be seen as something we 'do', but a part of 'being', which happens appropriately if we learn how to use ourselves well. It is interesting that when a person inhibits and gives directions, one of the most common results is a natural expansion in the breathing. This occurs simply as a result of an improvement in the primary control. Alexander teachers work with students to improve their use, and one aspect of improved functioning that results is an improvement in the breathing mechanisms, greater freedom in the ribs and diaphragm, and a release in all the muscles of the larynx, allowing freedom and control in the voice.

Fig. 6.8

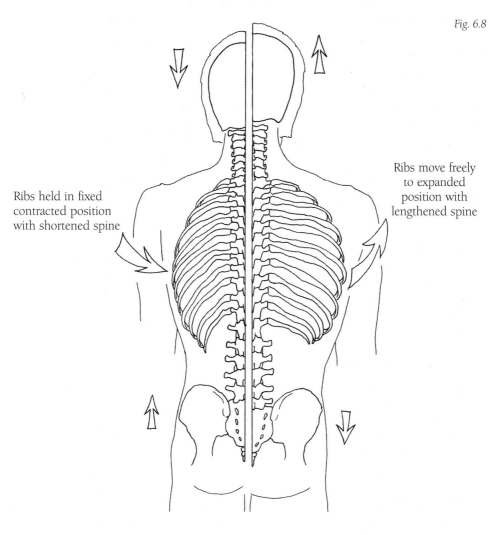

Ribs held in fixed contracted position with shortened spine

Ribs move freely to expanded position with lengthened spine

Widening the Ribs

Using the Voice

As the use of a person changes, so does the tone of voice. Our voice is an expression of the whole self, just as our movements are. As the muscles of the larynx release, and the breathing becomes freer, the sounds we produce reflect these changes, and they have a richer, more integrated quality. This applies to the speaking and singing voice, and using the technique in the training of actors and singers has resulted in great improvements in vocal abilities.

The subtle relationship between the head, neck, and back can either enhance the functioning of the body as a whole, or if it is not working well it can interfere with good functioning. In most people today that relationship, the primary control, is not working well and so their use is constantly acting against their good functioning.

Chapter Seven

Thinking in Activity

It is therefore obvious that the correct order of procedure for teacher and pupil is first for the pupil to learn to prevent himself from doing the wrong things which cause the imperfections or defects, and then, as a secondary consideration in procedure, to learn the correct way to use the mental and physical mechanisms concerned. (FMA,MSI)

Alexander experimented until he found an optimum arrangement for the head and neck, but when he tried to maintain this new balance, during reciting, or movement, he found the force of habit took over and the old mis-uses returned. He had to discover a means whereby he could maintain the primary control without interference during movement or speech, and so bring about an improved use of the self, and it was through the combined thought processes of inhibition and direction that the solution to this dilemma lay.

Working with our thoughts to bring about changes is a very powerful technique and a very popular one today. There are many systems which do this, such as positive thinking, affirmations, creative visualization and self-hypnosis, and they can be very effective. Alexander was very suspicious of these methods because he believed they were based on faulty sensory experience, and because they did not develop conscious control. Nevertheless, his technique of thinking in activity has similarities with other systems, in that they all recognise that thinking certain thoughts can be an extremely powerful and effective means of creating changes in the whole person, by counteracting habitual reactive behaviour.

One important way in which his technique differs from others is that it is based upon the process of inhibition. Inhibition comes before giving directions, and it is the directions which are similar to other forms of positive thinking. Alexander's technique involved a two-pronged attack on his habitual responses. Firstly he stopped the desire to 'do' anything. In this way he was inhibiting the excitation of the nervous system from going into an automatic reaction. Secondly he gave directions to himself which consisted of a positive alternative to the habitual use. Only these two activities carried out persistently, and at the same time, made it possible for fundamental change to occur.

Inhibition

Inhibition is a physiological process which operates in all animals. It is the capacity of the organism to not react to a stimulus. Our nervous systems operate on a stimulus-response basis. The neural messages are transmitted to the muscles, via the motor neurons, and there are two and only two possible messages, excitation and inhibition. In fact the muscles are receiving excitatory and inhibitory messages all the time, and it is only when the excitatory impulse builds to a sufficiently high level that muscular activity takes place. Our nervous systems are constantly bombarded with stimuli and if we were unable to inhibit reactions to all these stimuli our behaviour would be totally dis-coördinated. Spasticity is an example of a nervous system in which there is too little inhibitory response, and so the musculature is engaged in dis-coördinated uncontrolled reactivity. In a normal nervous system the inhibitory response to stimuli is dominant and only when the excitation becomes very powerful do the inhibitory mechanisms give way to the excitatory ones.

The physiological function of inhibition is to allow any animal to organise itself to respond in a co-ordinated and integrated way to a stimulus. The excitatory response to any stimulus creates tension and shortening in the muscles, particularly in the muscles that connect the head to the neck. This is as true of animals as it is of humans. The inhibitory response creates lengthening and strengthening in the musculature, and particularly in the head-neck muscles. And so inhibition as an unconscious physiological process brings about a freeing and lengthening in the neck muscles and an improvement in the Primary Control.

Alexander reasoned that because of the nature of the modern world, civilized human beings have been subjected to much greater and increasing excitation of the nervous system in the last several hundred years than in the previous several million years, when the rate of change of human society was relatively slow. Because of this, our natural inhibitory mechanisms are not functioning sufficiently well to allow for co-ordinated and integrated behaviour, in the face of increased excitation. In order to balance this situation we have to take conscious control of our inhibitory mechanism in order to encourage the natural freeing and lengthening response in the head and neck, and therefore throughout the body, to occur. We have to help our nervous systems to function better. Inhibiting a reaction to a stimulus means simply not responding, neither reacting, nor resisting reaction which is also a form of reaction.

Inhibition should become a part of our continuous thinking process. There are times for instance, during stress and excitation, when it is more advantageous than others, but ideally it needs to be cultivated as a conscious habit which influences all our behaviour. Sometimes it is a momentary pause in preparation for action. At other times that momentary inhibition may be in response to some unwelcome request, and instead of reacting automatically we may say 'I'd like time to think about this', and so we can create a longer inhibitory pause before reacting to a stimulus. Lying in semi-supine is an act of inhibition. It takes us out of our habitual situation and creates a space in which releases can occur, in which the inhibitory mechanisms can return to balance, and it does it in a physical position which is most advantageous for those releases. Inhibition in this sense is not to be confused with the repressive fixing that Freud called 'Inhibition'. It is essentially a freeing mechanism, a physiological function which improves the muscle tone of the body, and frees the mind and body for more conscious creative activity.

If use is the foundation of the technique, inhibition is the fulcrum around which it moves. Without inhibition the entire attempt to change one's habitual behaviour becomes quite redundant and meaningless. Learning consciously to inhibit gives us the possibility of freedom from the slavery of our neuro-muscular response system. It means we can begin to operate from choice and not from habit. And this was why Alexander saw his technique as having evolutionary significance. It was the opportunity for man to take control of his destiny in a meaningful way. For if we can successfully say 'no' to those habitual mental and muscular responses, which dis-coördinate us and destroy our functional integration, perhaps we will in time be able to take control of the disintegrative, destructive and negative patterns that are a habitual part of the social mechanism, and which roll on relentlessly towards the destruction of the planet.

• *Games of Inhibition* •

Doings — Choose one of your habitual activities, such as sitting down, writing, or talking to people, and practise for a day having a moment's inhibition before you move into that activity. And so for a day you may remember to pause for a moment and let everything quieten down, every time you are about to sit down. Simply decide not to sit down for a moment. See how easy you find it to do this, and notice the effect it has upon you. On another day you may decide to inhibit before standing up, and on another, before speaking. Experiment with different activities in order to learn about your own habitual responses. Working with the Alexander technique, inhibition is a constant process, and a difficult one to cultivate. Begin by choosing one simple everyday activity to work with. You may find you really enjoy it!

Sounds — List all the sounds that you are subjected to in an average day in your life, sounds like the telephone ringing, traffic noise, the radio or television, voices of other people, sounds of machinery. Take each sound in turn and recall it, and see if you can detect your physical, mental and emotional responses to that sound. They may be quite subtle, such as slightly increased tension in the shoulders, or they may be quite gross, like leaping up to answer the phone. Make a note of the sounds which seem to upset your balance most. Next time you hear those sounds, get in touch with all the neuromuscular responses, so you are as aware as you can be of the effect of that sound upon you. Then practise inhibition. Encourage your nervous system to not react, or to let go of its reaction.

Oughts — Recall situations in your life where you have felt pressured to 'do' something. Times when you have said to yourself, 'I really ought to do this but I don't want to'. Notice all the sensory responses that accompany the internal conflict. Experiment with saying 'No' to the pressure, creating a space where you can look more calmly at the situation and come to reasoned response. Notice the sensory changes that occur in your body as a result of saying 'No', even if it is only in your imagination.*

Direction

Another difficulty which pupils make for themselves is in connexion with the giving of guiding orders or directions. They speak sometimes as if it were a strange and new thing to ask them to give themselves orders, forgetting that they have been doing this subconsciously from their earliest days, else they would not be able to stand up without help, much less move about. (FMA, *CCC*)

Inhibition is the skill of being able to pause before responding to a stimulus. It is the ability to say 'No' when all your mental or physical or emotional habits are urging you into action. It is the ability to create a space so that the response need not be an automatic habitual one. And into that empty space, in which your nervous system is releasing muscular, mental and emotional tension, Alexander placed his 'Directions'.

---

* Our emotional responses are very complicated, and it is here that the confusion between Alexander's use of the word 'Inhibition' and Freud's use of the same word is at its greatest. I shall look at inhibition in relation to emotional responses in Part 2 of this book.

'Directions' are not something new that Alexander dreamed up. He realised that we direct our actions all the time, but that these directions are so automatic that we are not even aware that we are doing them. Whenever we move, our minds 'direct' what movements we are going to make. We mentally decide to sit or stand or walk or talk and then put that decision into practise. These directions are very vague compared to the detailed instructions that Alexander devised and called 'directions' but they are based on the same principle, that our mind instructs our body prior to voluntary movement.

Alexander devised directions for the use of his body which, as a result of experimentation and reasoning, he discovered would allow the body to operate in a better way. The directions are given to counteract the habitual misuse, so the first direction he gave was 'that the neck be free', simply to allow any undue muscular tension in the muscles of the neck to release. The second direction was that 'the head go forwards and up', which is precisely the opposite to the habitual tendency to pull the head back and down. And the third direction was 'that the back lengthen and widen', to counteract the tendency of shortening and narrowing in the back. The directions are not new and different actions, but counter-actions to the habitual wrong doings. They reinforce the inhibitory mechanisms which would bring about the same conditions. The directions are there to facilitate that process. In the last analysis the directions are a form of inhibition.

Alexander also insisted that the directions are all related to each other, they are not separate instructions. He saw giving the directions as a combined activity and suggested that a student say them 'all together, one after the other'. And so the primary directions are usually stated as a continuous series of orders as follows;

Free the neck, and allow the head to go forwards and up, in such a way that the back lengthens and widens.

Alexander arrived at these directions by reasoning out how to counteract the major misuses. These directions encourage the best functioning of the primary control. In addition Alexander employed other directions which related to other parts of the body, such as the arms or the knees, and directions that would be specific to the particular misuse pattern of each individual pupil, but these directions must never take over from the primary directions. The relationship of the head to the neck must be maintained in a good way as the other directions are given. All the directions should be seen as a whole, with the three primary directions leading the rest, just as the head leads the body. The body is a whole, much more than a collection of parts, and any change in one part of the body will affect the rest of the body. This concept of unity and wholeness is fundamental, and when we talk about the use of the self, we mean the whole self, for the way in which we move a part, such as an arm or a leg, will affect the whole self, and should be considered an action of the whole self. Therefore every movement of the body is affected by the primary control, and how well that is functioning.

Like inhibiting, directing is a thinking process. A direction is a preparation for doing and a method in which the doing can take place. It is a mental act of wishing, willing, wanting or ordering. Sometimes he called the directions 'orders'. They are instructions to the nervous system, but because they are not designed to bring about muscular shortening but muscular lengthening, they cannot be 'doings', as I explained in the Chapter 'How Muscles Work'. They are not exercises except in so much as they are mental exercises. However, when one is 'doing', that is moving or acting in some way, one still continues to direct, and provided the old habitual wrong 'doing' does not take over the activity, one is then said to be moving 'with direction' and this is the beginning of improved use.

• *Giving the Directions to your Mirror Image* •

Stand in front of the mirror, or preferably use two mirrors so you can see a side view as well. Stand with your feet hip-width apart, the weight falling evenly over the inside and outside of the foot, and with very slightly more weight on the heel than on the front of the foot.

Begin by pausing, stopping, inhibiting, allowing the nervous system to calm down. Simply look at your image in the mirror. Get in touch with your sensory awareness of how your body feels in that position. Notice all you can that is going on at a sensory level. Notice what thoughts and feelings you are having as you watch yourself in the mirror. If these thoughts and feelings are disturbing your equilibrium, pause and inhibit once more. Allow the information to come and go, and not to excite you. You may need to work at this for some time. Remember that you are not going to 'do' anything. You are simply working with your thoughts.

When you feel calm and centred, look at the image in the mirror and think your directions to the image. This is a good way of not allowing the directing to become a 'doing'.

Think to the image in the mirror that you want the neck of that image to be free, and the head to be releasing forwards and up. Remember that the purpose in directing is to encourage muscular release, and lengthening. If you try to do the directions you will be creating shortening and tension, the opposite of what you want.

Watch the image in the mirror. You may be quite surprised at how it changes in very subtle ways.

Now tell the image that the head should be releasing forwards and up in such a way that the back can lengthen and widen. Imagine this lengthening and widening process happening in your spine and ribs and throughout your body. Once again notice how thinking this and directing it at the image in the mirror may be producing some interesting subtle changes. It doesn't matter if you don't notice anything. The important thing is to not try to make the changes by doing things with your body. You are sending directing thoughts to it by means of the image in the mirror.

Continue to work with inhibition and direction of the primary directions for some time, watching your image in the mirror and going through the three directions one by one, all at the same time. Avoid stiffening the body or getting into a fixed position. If that seems to be happening go for a short walk around the room and then return to the mirror and continue to inhibit and direct.

You have been experimenting with the major directions Alexander taught his pupils in order to bring about an improvement in the primary control. They constitute a positive alternative to the major misuse pattern that we get into. A lot of people do not understand directions as a means of countering habitual misuse and so once more they get into 'doing' the directions which can only create shortening of the muscles involved. Often students think they are directing, whereas in fact they are getting into a fix, a rigid state, which is their 'idea' of what directing is. It is terribly difficult not to fall into these traps, when you are working on your own, which is why I constantly recommend, if you have never worked with an Alexander teacher, that you find a teacher to monitor what you are doing when directing and to help you understand your own perceptions of what is happening.

If you have worked with an Alexander teacher you will probably have used many additional directions to the ones here. Every teacher is different and so is every student, and to go into more detail is beyond the scope of this book.

Choice

Taking Inhibition and Direction into action – if we choose to
Thinking in activity by means of inhibition and direction allows us to move beyond the automatic activity of habit. Conscious control of the use of the self allows for a free-

dom of choice that was hitherto subtly denied to us. When we consciously inhibit we create a space in which choice can operate. Alexander brought this opportunity to choose into his experiments with reciting, and this new element eventually helped the experiments to be successful. His method was as follows.

1. Inhibit the habitual response to the stimulus (eg. to recite)

2. Give the new directions, all together, one after the other.

3. Continue to inhibit the old behaviour, and the old preparation for behaviour until one feels the new directions are being thought out strongly and clearly.

4. Continue to inhibit the stimulus to recite and in that space choose whether to:
   a. Recite.
   b. Do something quite different to reciting, such as lifting the hand up.
   c. Do nothing.

By creating a choice at this moment Alexander was able to avoid end-gaining. Whichever of the three options he chose, he chose firstly to maintain his good use in whatever he did. He took the attention off gaining his end, and put it onto maintaining the correct means for gaining the end. This meant that in time he was able to successfully recite while maintaining his improved use. He was able to take the directions into activity.

It was by intervening in the automatic response of the nervous system right up to the last possible moment while giving directions that continued through and beyond that last moment, that Alexander successfully changed his use. It was a long, laborious task, but the rewards were equal to the task, for he had learnt a control of the nervous system which up until then was unknown to Western man. And the effect of that control was greater freedom in mind and body, and the possibility of real choice at a fundamental level. He then was able to teach that freedom to others. And many who have been taught by him and by the teachers trained in his method realize that these skills are far-reaching in their potential. The world we live in is too busy, too full of excitatory stimulus. It is a world preoccupied with 'doing' and out of touch with 'being'. Inhibition allows us to contact our being nature, to pause and examine what we are doing, thinking, feeling. Inhibition brings us back to our centre, so that our actions come from a calm balanced centre inside ourselves, not a nervous excited response to something outside ourselves. Then direction and choice move us into action once more, with the possibility of a new improved use of the self.

Constructive Conscious Control

Just as our movement is better when we lead with the head, so we need to lead with our reason, our conscious awareness. The information of the senses is absolutely essential to good functioning, and to personal integration, but while we use that information to help us in our choices, we make our choices from our reasoning. This is not a dictatorship, with the mind ruling the sensory nature to the point of ruling it out. It is a co-operative system with both aspects of the self playing an important part. When we inhibit we give ourselves an opportunity to really assess what is happening at a sensory level. We can then choose to inhibit what is not helpful and direct what is helpful to us. Just as the head leads the body, so the conscious mind respectfully assesses the valuable information of the physical and emotional feelings, and makes judgements, leading the self into an increasingly integrated state. Every aspect of the self has an important role to play in living and expressing the whole person. The ability of human beings to move from instinctive habitual behaviour into conscious control was considered by Alexander to be an important step in our evolutionary development. Unfortunately because we live in a society that tends to repress feelings it may be difficult to accept a co-operative relationship between our feeling nature and our reasoning and I look at this in more detail in part two of this book.

• *Giving the Directions in Semi-Supine* •

Lie down in semi-supine and allow yourself to move into that quiet listening space, which is a form of inhibiting. Spend the first few minutes observing yourself in whatever way you want to so you are getting in touch with the information of your sensory mechanism.

When you feel calm in your mind and your body begin to think the primary directions:

1. Think that you want your neck to be free.

Tell yourself how free your neck is and use all the visual ideas that we worked with in Chapter Four to reinforce the attention and energy behind this direction. Imagine the Atlanto-occipital joint, and the vertebrae of the neck, the sub-occipital muscles, the larger muscles, and the larynx all releasing and allowing the neck to be free.

2. Think that your neck is free and so your head is moving 'forwards and out'.

Because you are lying with your head on books, and as long as the number of books is giving you a 'forwards' stimulus then the lengthening that occurs in this position is experienced as an outwards movement of the head away from the body.

3. Think that your neck is free and your head is moving outwards behind you in such a way that your back is lengthening and widening.

Visualize each vertebra of the spine releasing, the discs getting thicker and spongier and the muscles of the spine lengthening. Visualize the lengthening in the spine and the effect this has on separating the ribs, which can then move more freely, this in turn creating a widening throughout the torso.

4. Free the neck and send the head forwards and out in such a way that the back lengthens and widens, widening across the upper part of the arms.

This direction allows a widening to occur across the shoulder girdle, back and front. If you look at figure 7.1, you will see that the shoulder joints are the point on the skeleton where the arm connects to the torso. By directing the two upper parts of the arm away from each other this allows widening to occur across the chest, upper back and under the arms. This direction is very helpful for freeing the breathing as it allows much more space for the ribs to move.

Fig. 7.1

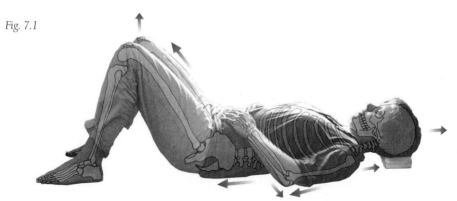

Skeletal structure of body in semi-supine, showing directions

5. Free the neck and send the head forwards and out in such a way that the back lengthens and widens, widening across the upper part of the arms and sending the knees forwards and away.

Because you are lying with your knees up and about hip width apart, the best way to work with this direction is to direct the knees upwards towards the ceiling. Just as the last direction allowed a widening and freeing in the shoulder girdle, so this direction allows a widening and freeing in the pelvic girdle. By sending the knees up towards the ceiling this encourages among other things, release of any tensions in the hip joints and lengthening in the muscles of the upper and lower legs. One of the effects of this direction is that as a result of releases in the legs there are releases in the diaphragm, which then allows the breathing mechanisms to work more freely.

These five directions cover the whole body, giving positive suggestions for how the arms and legs can integrate with the trunk of the body in addition to the lengthening, widening and freeing of the head, neck and back relationship.

When you come into standing you may like to stand in front of a mirror and continue to give the five directions, 'all together, one after the other', as Alexander would say, inhibiting your old habitual use, and encouraging an improved use of the self while standing.

The five directions when standing:

1. Let the neck be free....

2. And allow the head to be moving forwards and up....

3. In such a way that the back lengthens and widens....

4. Widening across the upper part of the arms....

5. And sending the knees forwards and away....

Chapter Eight

Interfering

As long as we adhere in everything we do to the principle of consciously inhibiting inter-ference with the employment of the primary control, then our ordinary daily activities can be made a constant means of psychophysical development in its fullest sense. (FMA, UCL)

The beauty of the Alexander Technique is that it combines the best of both worlds. It offers a 'return to grace', a co-ordinated organism, with a reliable sensory mechanism, and an advance to conscious control which leads us into a continuously more har-monious and integrated state. If we can use our conscious control to undo all the interferences that have created our poor posture and misuse, then poise and improved use, and a graceful way of moving and living will emerge. This is the pearl of great price which the Alexander technique can teach us: that we learn by unlearning, we 'do' by 'undoing', that when we stop doing the wrong thing the right thing does itself.

In order to improve our use we don't have to 'do' anything. We have to learn to 'undo' the things that are interfering with our natural potential for good use. Our habits cause the interferences. Because we habitually pull back the head, certain mus-cles of the neck and back have become habitually shortened and narrowed. We have to learn how to release that unnecessary muscle tension. We know how to create it - by 'doing' things, especially by pulling the head back. Learning how to inhibit and direct our nervous systems allows us to gain control over the 'undoing' part of our muscles, so they are able to release, and as they release they allow the primary control to function in a better way.

Endgaining and the 'Means Whereby'

Very frequently we are told that the cause of most of our difficulties is the increasing com-plexity of the demands of living in the present stage of civilization. It is much more to the point to say that our real difficulties arise from the almost universal adoption in practical life of the lowly evolved 'endgaining' principle in our attempts to meet these demands, the result being that we cultivate within ourselves a condition of stress and strain. (FMA, CCC)

The way we interfere most of all is by the habit of endgaining. Endgaining simply means acting directly to bring about a specific end, without due attention to the way in which we bring about that action. This habit is so much a part of all our experience, in our personal lives and in the world around us, it is almost impossible to conceive what living would be without it. 'The ends justifies the means' is a saying of our times, which Alexander replaced by suggesting that we 'take care of the means and the ends will take care of themselves'.

Endgaining has to be understood in contrast to the concept of the 'means whereby'. Acting with attention to the means whereby, means that the primary aim is to maintain good use, a good primary control in all that we do, and that it is secondary what end we bring about with this good use. And so we approach our ends indirectly, giving our attention first and foremost to how we operate. By operating with due attention to the means whereby, everything we do is contributing to our health and well-being, and the chances are that we will be much more successful in achieving our ends, because we are operating from a reasoned approach and a correct means whereby we gain them.

The key to maintaining the means whereby, and therefore not endgaining, is inhibition. It is only by a continuous process of inhibiting the many mental and physical habits that interfere with good use that we can stop endgaining and operate with good use in all that we do. Endgaining comes in many shapes and sizes, all habits of mind and body which interfere with good use.

Doing

We nearly always pull our heads back, and indeed misuse ourselves in many other ways, in order to do something. All our daily activities, from sitting, standing, walking, writing, speaking, singing and so on tend to be done in a way that interferes with good use, unless we approach them by giving our attention to the way in which we do them, rather than simply getting them done. Even when we intellectually understand this it doesn't necessarily mean we will operate any better, because learning to inhibit the endgaining habits is a long and challenging process. Nevertheless we do have the possibility of changing. As soon as we learn to recognize what we are doing wrong, we have choice. We can continue in the habitual endgaining way or we can learn to pay attention to the means whereby, and begin to misuse ourselves less.

Alexander spent a long time standing in front of the mirror, inhibiting, then giving directions, and then thinking about reciting. At the thought of reciting, all sorts of 'neuromuscular preparations' could be subtly detected as the old habitual response pattern surfaced. This was his endgaining - wanting to do the reciting rather than wanting to maintain the means whereby of the new directions he was giving himself. By saying 'no' to all the neuromuscular responses that the thought of reciting stimulated, he was removing the interferences to a better use of himself.

Often when a student is giving directions he is 'doing' them. That is, instead of inhibiting the old habits and just thinking of the new direction, the student will try to make it happen. So he will really try to widen the shoulders, for example, by a movement of the muscles. If the student is preoccupied with having wide shoulders in the front of the body he will tighten the shoulder blades at the back and cause a seeming widening at the front, or if the student is wanting a broad backed look to the shoulders he will tighten in the chest area, hollowing the chest and pushing the back out to make it seem wider. Sending the head forwards and up becomes a gentle push and so on. Each of these 'doing' attempts interferes with the possibility of improved use of the self. The directions cannot be 'done', as they are in themselves a way of undoing muscle tension, and so this 'doing' interference is just adding another layer of muscle tension on top of what is already there.

Fixing

Often a student has a good experience and he doesn't want to lose it so the musculature tightens around the position that felt good. What was a beautifully free neck then becomes a stiff and rigid neck, in more or less the same position, but having totally lost the quality of freedom and lengthening that it had before. Or the teacher has created a lengthening and widening in the back which the student wants to maintain, so the student puts a 'muscular clamp' onto it, which naturally has exactly the opposite effect to the end he wanted to gain. This 'holding on', or 'fixing', is another form of endgaining.

Often we respond to stress by 'fixing' a muscular pattern so that the muscles are unable to release. This particularly happens with breathing. When we 'hold our breath', we actually hold onto our rib cages and diaphragms, among other things. Fixing occurs when we feel unsafe. Our muscles hold on. They go into a fix. Change can be very frightening, and our response to it can be to be as fixed and unchanging as we can be in our bodies. As we learn to inhibit the fixing and become more flexible in our minds and bodies we will be able to flow more easily with the inevitable changes of life.

We often fix our muscles if we want to hold ourselves in a certain position, but this fixing is quite unnecessary. It is using an increased amount of muscle tension to create the posture. It is not getting the maximum output from the minimum effort. Sometimes a student tries to stop pulling the head back by fixing it firmly in what they think is a 'forwards and up' position. This simply creates harmful tension in the neck muscles which interferes with the primary control. Alexander Teachers are very wary of being described as people who improve posture, because the word posture suggests a position and has a fixedness and rigidity about it, all the things we are working against.

Fixed ideas can interfere enormously with a process of changing. If a person has a conviction about what is right for him, or what he can or can't do, it can be very difficult to create an experience in contradiction to that fixed expectation. Our mental habits of thought interfere with our good use, just as much as our unconscious habitual behaviour. Alexander believed that they were the greatest stumbling block:

Certain of these fixed ideas are encountered in the case of almost every pupil; fixed ideas, for example, as to what constitutes the right and what the wrong method of going to work as a pupil; fixed ideas in regard to the necessity for concentration, if success is to attend the efforts of pupil and teacher; also a fixed belief, (based on subconscious guidance) that if a pupil is corrected for a defect, he should be taught to do something in order to correct it, instead of being taught, as a first principle how to prevent (inhibition) the wrong thing from being done . . . I have no hesitation in stating that the pupil's fixed ideas and conceptions are the cause of the major part of his difficulties. (FMA, CCC)

Emotional Attitudes

Students of the technique come up against their endgaining all the time, in many different guises. Wanting to please the teacher, or wanting to get it right, or being afraid of getting it wrong, are powerful ways of interfering. Emotional anxiety adds a whole new layer of tension to the situation and interferes with the primary control. The fear reflexes in the body are stimulated, which creates shortening in the muscles of the neck and throughout the body. As Alexander put it, 'I don't want you to give a damn if you're right or not. Directly you don't care if you're right or not, the impeding obstacle is gone.'

It's terribly difficult not to endgain, because we all want results. No-one wants to feel they are wasting their time. I am not suggesting that we should not want results. Ends, or goals, are a very necessary part of life, but goals must be balanced by a commitment to the moment, to living in the present. We probably all know people who are quite unable to stop, because they have so much to do. They organize their life entirely around visible results, and never leave any space for just being alive. The quality of life of these people is often appalling, but they are so out of touch with themselves and their needs that they are unlikely to be aware of this until there is a crisis, either in their health, or in their personal lives which can no longer stand the pace of this endgaining existence. You do not score many points on the social value scale for enjoying living in the here and now, but those people who have managed to bypass the rat race and learned to take care of the means whereby of living, know that it has its own rewards. It is not that they no longer have any goals, but that part of those goals is that the process of achieving them is fulfiling and life-enhancing rather than life-destructive.

Endgaining is the great villain in the Alexander Drama. It crops up time and time again in subtler and subtler ways, and it is a principle on which, not only do we lead our personal lives, but the social and political world conducts its affairs, a deeply entrenched cultural habit. For the end of profit, wars have been fought, rainforests have been desecrated, rivers and seas have been polluted. In opposition to this the Alexander principle attempts to weave a totally new way of being, in which the 'how' of what we do becomes primary, and the end, secondary.

There are interferences to good use which cannot be called endgaining, because they are quite lacking in any intention, such as when we pull our heads back as a reflex response which I described as the startle response pattern. In principle this should not be serious because the reflex occurs and then releases, so the shortening of the muscles is momentary. The problem is that this reflex response has become habitual and fixed in many people. Inhibition and direction over a period of time will allow this reflex response to 'undo' and the muscles of the neck to release so that the primary control is not interfered with. However if this has become fixed it will take some time for the muscles to return to a released state.

There are other interferences to good use that cannot always be dealt with using the methods of the Alexander technique alone. Sometimes, past traumatic experiences, mental, emotional and physical, become locked in the structure of the body and cannot be released without help from a specialist in this field. There may be other problems due to diet or illness that need special attention, and cannot be related purely and simply to misuse. Often old traumas are released by continued application of the technique, but not always, and then I would advise people to find therapists who can help them with their specific problems. The Alexander technique creates a general change in conditions in a person, as a result of which many specific problems go away, but it does not focus on specific problems as such.

• *Inhibiting the Interferences* •

The way to stop interfering with the primary control is through inhibition. As soon as you are aware enough to recognise an interference you can inhibit it. You may need the help of a teacher to point out ways in which you are interfering, and help you develop your self-awareness, but you will be able to observe some of your habits yourself. Refining one's self awareness reveals layer upon layer of interferences, which is why the potential for improvement goes on and on.

In the next exercise, once again you have the opportunity to work on yourself in the way that Alexander did, but with a clearer picture of all the interferences that you may have to inhibit.

Stand in front of the mirror. Look at your image and pause. Inhibit all the excitatory stimulus that you are aware of, both physical, emotional and mental.

Inhibit the tendency to pull the head back and down.

Inhibit the tendency to make standing a 'doing'. Just be standing.

Inhibit the tendency to 'fix' in the standing position. Think of yourself as quite soft and flexible.

Give directions to the image in the mirror to 'free the neck and allow the head to go forwards and up in such a way that the back lengthens and widens'.

Inhibit the tendency to 'do' or 'fix' the directions. If you feel you are getting fixed, and you cannot release this by inhibiting, you may need to go for a short walk around the room before returning to the mirror and beginning the whole process again. Inhibit the desire to 'get it right'.

Inhibit the anxiety of 'trying'.

Inhibit all the judgmental voices inside you, telling you you are a born failure and couldn't free your neck if you had six Alexander teachers helping you.

Inhibit any other unhelpful thoughts, and physical interferences.

Give your directions again.

Inhibit any other thoughts or feelings or muscular responses that interfere with the free flowing of the new directions. Now think about speaking a sentence or two, to your image in the mirror.

Notice all the neuromuscular responses that come up when you think about speaking. Observe these in as much detail as you can, both kinaesthetically and visually.

Say to yourself that you are not going to speak.

Inhibit the reactive thoughts, feelings, fixings and doings that occurred when you decided to speak.

Return to simply standing looking at your image in the mirror, giving your directions, and inhibiting all the mental and physical interferences.

Consider speaking a sentence or two, and inhibit all the interfering reactions to that idea.

Continue to inhibit the stimulus to speak and choose what to do next:

  a) Recite
  b) Raise a hand
  c) Do nothing

Keep inhibiting and directing as you choose which alternative to move into.

Whichever option you choose, your primary concern is to maintain the correct means whereby, and so if you move or speak, you will be doing so 'with direction'. Observe yourself carefully to see if the old habits reappear. And so on . . .

This exercise should give you some idea of how slowly and patiently Alexander worked on his voice problem:

> *I would give the new directions in front of the mirror for long periods together, for successive days and weeks and sometimes even months, without attempting to 'do' them.* (FMA,UOS)

It is significant that he evolved his technique through careful study of himself in mirrors, because mirrors tend to stimulate lots of excitatory responses and fear reflexes, and to refuse to respond to those stimuli one must be a master of inhibition, which is what Alexander taught himself to be. After all, when you look at a mirror it is the closest you ever get to really facing yourself. In the second part of this book there are more mirror exercises, which deal with the responses that come up in this subtle self-observatory work.

Chapter Nine

Working with a Teacher

I am not interested in the particular manifestation of a person's wrongness. I do the same thing for every one, whether he comes to me with flat feet or nervous tension. I help him to get his Primary Control working again, and when this happens the pupil will be on the right total pattern and his use and functioning will be at their potential best. (FMA)

So far in this book I have described how Alexander worked out for himself the principles and evolution of his technique. As far as I know he is the only person who learned the technique in this way. Most people learn by studying with a teacher who is trained to teach the Alexander technique. This method is much easier and less time consuming, and it is the one Alexander himself recommended. It is a valuable part of the learning process to go through the experiments Alexander made, as I have done in this book, but to use this method alone would require great dedication and persistence, qualities which Alexander certainly possessed.

When Alexander began to take pupils and teach his technique to others he would tell his pupils what to do, what to think, and so on. When he was working with pupils in movement he would guide them with his hands; and it was then he discovered that his pupils learnt much more from the guidance and contact of his hands than from the verbal instructions he gave them. Because Alexander had worked patiently for years to bring his own organism into balance and co-ordination, he found his hands could transmit co-ordinating signals to the nervous system of the pupil, signals which encouraged inhibition, release and good direction and so brought about an improvement in the primary control of the person he was working on. By simply placing his hands upon a pupil, and at the same time maintaining his own primary control and good use, the muscles in the neck of the pupil would release, the head would go forwards and up and the back would lengthen and widen.

In addition Alexander could feel with his hands what was happening in the musculature of his pupil, where he was tightening or fixing or interfering in some other way. And so he began to teach by using his hands to give the pupil a totally new experience

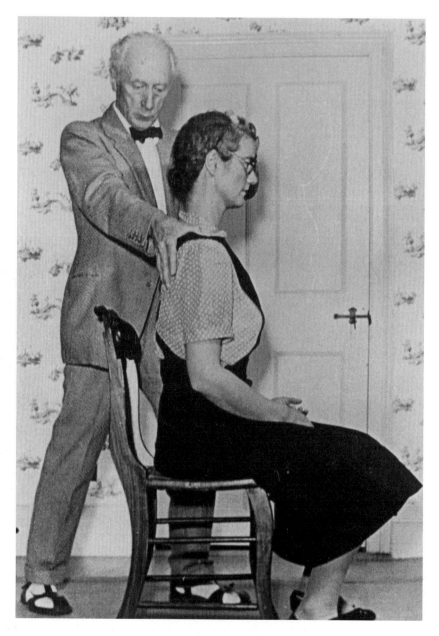

F. M. Alexander teaching

of the primary control working well without interference. To begin with, this experience would be momentary and at best would not last much longer than the length of the lesson. But in time the pupil would learn to maintain the new use for longer until eventually he could maintain the new use independently of Alexander. Later, other people trained with Alexander to teach his technique, by working on their own coordination and use very thoroughly for three years until their own use was extremely good and their sensory mechanisms were once again reliable and so they too were able to use their hands in this way.

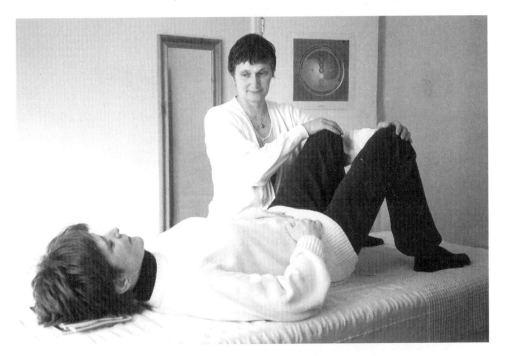

Teacher (the author) working with a student in the semi-supine position

Learning the principles of the Alexander technique with a teacher is a much more reliable and efficient method than working it out for oneself because when a person is working on her own the only way of judging when she is doing something correctly and when she is interfering with the primary control is by watching her actions in a mirror. She cannot rely upon her feelings to judge what is right, because they are unreliable while her use is unreliable. And so the observational skills must be very keen

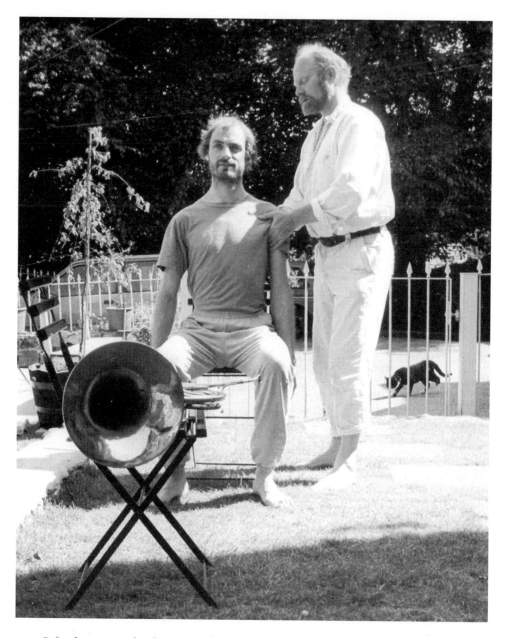

Before learning to play the French Horn with good use, the student simply learns to sit well

and acute to detect minute and subtle movements that may be interfering with good use. The Alexander teacher is trained to observe visually those very subtle changes and to 'listen' with her hands, in addition to giving an experience of improved co-ordination, so she can help the student experience the neurophysiological changes that come about with an improved use of the self. Nevertheless we must be grateful that Alexander was prepared to persist in the slow process of re-education in the use of the self without the help of an expert or he would never have evolved his technique and passed it on to others.

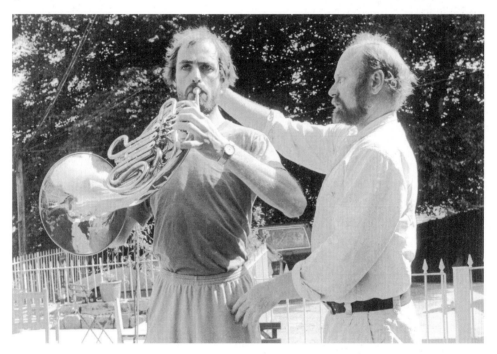

Learning how to play a musical instrument with good use

Most Alexander teachers in this country teach the Alexander technique by giving a series of lessons to a student. On average a person needs a minimum of twenty to thirty lessons in order to be able to maintain a level of good use independently of a teacher. Some teachers also teach groups of people in addition to giving private lessons, and some teachers, mainly in America, do all their teaching in groups. There are advantages and disadvantages to both types of teaching. In a group situation the students are able to develop and refine their visual awareness because they are able to observe each other. Also they are in a much better position to understand those problems that we all have in common in our mental and physical habits, and other problems that are unique to each individual. For example, we all tend to pull the head back, but not all of us hold the shoulders forwards. Mentally, we all tend to be very poor at inhibiting but some people get much more anxious than others about whether they are right or wrong. In a group situation similarities and differences can be discussed and clarified and this can lead to a greater understanding of our interferences, and of the principles in general.

The disadvantage of group work is that the members of the group do not get as much individual attention as they would in a private lesson, and this individual attention is essential for the student to experience changes in her use. When a teacher works individually, in one lesson she may want a student to lie in semi-supine on the table while she works on her in order to release the overcontractions in the musculature. With another student or in another lesson the teacher may want to teach the student how to move from standing to sitting. She may give a lot of attention to detailed directions that might not be appropriate with another student. We are all unique although we do share major misuses in common with each other. With one person it might be appropriate to think of freeing the jaw at the same time as freeing the neck, with another it might be more important to think of releasing in the knees or in the toes. Although the purpose of the work is always the same, to bring about an improvement in the primary control, every individual requires an individual approach and it is difficult to give this in any depth in a group situation. A combination of group work and individual work is ideal for learning the technique but not always possible to arrange.

What a student experiences during a course of Alexander work differs enormously from person to person. Some people feel energized, light and free, right from the start, while others feel quite heavy and exhausted to begin with and want to go to bed and rest, and other people don't feel very much at all and wonder what it's all about. Some people have a very emotional response to the work. It brings up feelings of sadness or alternatively bliss. Some people feel an awful lot on their first lesson and other people feel very little until they have had several lessons. Some people find their pains have disappeared and others find they ache all over. Some people feel as though they have grown and are enormous and others feel very weak and vulnerable. It can be bewildering for a student because although the teacher appears to be doing virtually nothing at all, a lot of changes take place. The nervous system of the student is assimilating a lot of new information as a result of the gentle contact of the teacher's hands. An Alexander teacher does not manipulate in the way an osteopath or a masseur does.

She simply places her hands on the student, inhibits and gives directions with her mind, and these signals are transmitted through her hands. When she is working on movement she will guide the student through the movement in a way that does not interfere with the primary control of herself or her student.

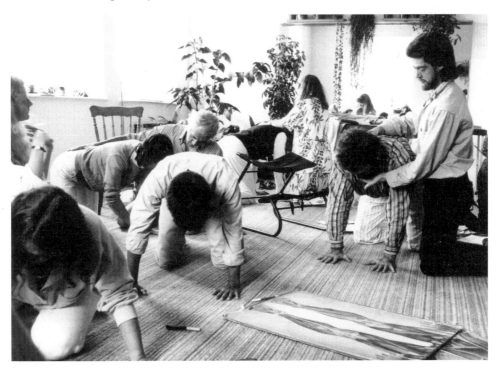

Group work – crawling with good use strengthens the back

Probably the first experience most students feel is the experience of inhibition although they may not realise that that is what it is. The system calms down, the student feels more centred and less excitable. Later she may feel the directions working through her body and have the sense that she is 'going up' as her neck frees and the primary control begins to work better. This upward flow can be felt throughout the body and gives a sense of lightness and freedom. Usually it is accompanied by unexpected releasing breaths as the ribs open and the breathing mechanisms are stimulated into more expansive activity resulting in the widening of the torso. But for many students these light upward feelings which are the hallmark of the technique are not experienced for a long time. As Lessons continue, the experience of inhibition and the directions working through the body, and the resulting improvement in the primary control, becomes more consistent. Students are able to maintain the conditions for themselves for longer periods. Usually improvements in functioning become notice-able, aches and pains fade away, and posture and movement improves.

If you are working with an Alexander teacher or are about to start then the best advice I can give is not to have any expectations about how the lessons will affect you, but to be very interested and curious as to how they do. What you are embarking upon is a process of getting to know yourself in quite a new and different way, and one of the first things to notice is how you respond to the lessons. It is well worthwhile keeping a notebook and jotting down the things you have noticed. The effects of an Alexander lesson may carry on for several hours after the lesson, sometimes for the next few days. It will be interesting to compare the differences between earlier and later lessons. Also see if you can separate your responses into different categories:

Sensations: Physical sensations you noticed during and after your lesson (eg. tingling in the legs/headache goes etc.).

Emotions: Notice how you respond emotionally to the work. (eg. happiness, sadness, cynicism, irritation, assertiveness, peacefulness).

Thoughts: Notice any thoughts and images you have during and after the lesson.

Do not feel upset if you barely remember any responses - and if you do feel upset, make a note of that. What are you thinking about yourself that upsets you? Everything you notice helps you develop your self-awareness. Everyone is different and there is no 'right' way to react to the teaching. By making the decision to improve your use you are learning how to take care of yourself in the best possible way, and so it will help if you observe your responses sympathetically. If you feel tired after a lesson accept the helpful information your body is giving you and allow yourself to rest.

Learning to operate with good use cannot happen overnight. An Alexander teacher will help you to see what your habitual misuses are, and give you an experience of operating without them. She will teach you how to inhibit the interferences that are causing the misuses and to give directions for a new improved use. When you begin to understand your misuses, and to inhibit them and give directions for a new improved use, you don't move immediately from misuse to perfect use. You begin the slow careful work of improvement and refinement. I hope that working with this book will help you in this process. To begin with you will need the help of the teacher to maintain the primary control for you, but in time you will find you are able to maintain these improved conditions for yourself and apply them to your daily life in many ways both mentally and physically. Eventually you will be able to take responsibility for your own good use without the help of a teacher. At this point you are making the Alexander technique your own, a real living part of your everyday life and I hope it will enrich your life as much as it has mine. Alexander looked forward to the day when Alexander teachers would become redundant because the human race as a whole had learnt how to operate with good use, passing these skills on to their children as a part of their upbringing:

I wish to do away with such teachers as I am myself. My place in the present economy is due to a misunderstanding of the causes of our present physical debility, and when this disability is finally eliminated the specialized practitioner will have no place, no uses. This may be a dream of the future, but in its beginnings it is now capable of realization. Every man, woman and child holds the possibility of physical perfection; it rests with each one of us to attain it by personal understanding and effort .

(FMA,MSI)

Chapter Ten

Fundamentals for Living

When once a reasonably adequate part of a new generation has become properly co-ordinated, we shall have assurance for the first time that men and women of the future will be able to stand on their own feet, equipped with satisfactory psycho-physical equilibrium, to meet with readiness, confidence, and happiness instead of fear, confusion, and discontent, the buffetings and contingencies of their surroundings. John Dewey (Intro. *CCC*)

The Alexander technique with its mixture of simplicity and subtle complexity offers the human race a remedy for a situation which is rapidly deteriorating. It suggests that we look at the way in which we do things, and it shows us that there is a way of doing everything which is life-enhancing and truly delightful. It is both simple and immediate, yet profound and far-reaching in its implications. It is not the sort of remedy that you take from a bottle, and expect a miraculous cure. The remedy involves time and attention, the commitment to relearning the fundamentals of living. As one student said 'Oh, I see, this is a life-sentence!' That is quite an undertaking, but the technique offers a method that works, and the rewards are immeasurable, not only for the individual but for the human race as a whole. Alexander spent most of his long life teaching others his technique and letting the world know about the value of his discoveries. As a young man he had been inspired by Shakespeare's lines:

'What a piece of work is a man! how noble in reason! how infinite in faculty!
in form and moving how express and admirable! in action how like an angel!
in apprehension how like a god! the beauty of the world! the paragon of animals!'

Later when Alexander discovered how much we misuse ourselves, how unreliable our sensory appreciation is, and how we are ruled by our unconscious habits, he reconsidered these words. As he put it:

Opposite: *Alexander teacher and students learning to sit and stand well*

For what could be less 'noble in reason', less 'infinite in faculty' than that man despite his potentialities, should have fallen into such error in the use of himself and in this way brought about such a lowering in his standard of functioning that in everything he attempts to accomplish, these harmful conditions tend to become more and more exaggerated? (FMA, *UOS*)

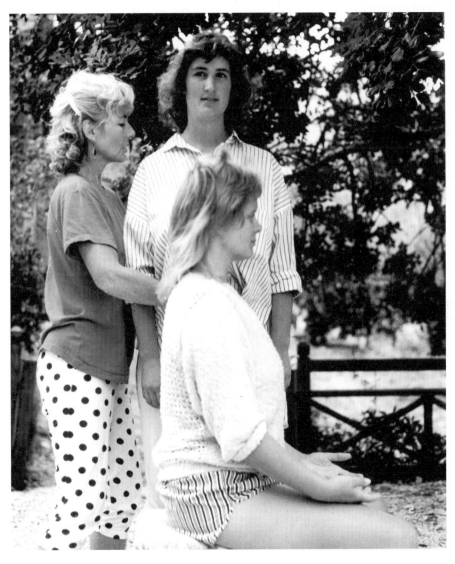

I remember hearing a story about a highly advanced Swami who visited this country and watched a lot of Yoga teachers doing their yoga postures. Afterwards he said 'Why don't you learn to do something simple, like sitting or standing, well.'

If we learn to operate well in the fundamentals of living, those simple activities of moving, breathing, talking, then how much greater is our potential for succeeding in more challenging and creative activities that develop from these fundamental ones. Alexander's teaching offers humanity a return to Shakespeare's vision. This is the gift offering of the Alexander technique; the possibility of an enriched experience in all areas of life.

Applying the Technique to Life

Whatever you do the technique can help the quality of your life to improve. It can help you to learn how to sit, stand, move, write, drive, think, and feel in richer and freer ways. The technique is a foundation for living, and it comes to life through being applied to the daily activities of life. It offers both a mental and physical approach to all activity, and a method of bringing about changes which can be applied to all aspects of life. It does not only offer the solution to the problem of our use, it gives the 'means whereby' we can change our use, careful moment by moment procedures, which are the Art of Changing. These procedures can be applied to much more than our physical use and I develop these ideas in Part Two of this book. To conclude Part One of the book there is a diagrammatic summary of the fundamental concepts of the Alexander Technique.

The adoption of conscious guidance and control (man's supreme inheritance) must follow, and the outcome will be a race of men and women who will outstrip their ancestors in every known sphere, and enter new spheres as yet undreamt of by the great majority of the civilized peoples of our time. The world will then make in one century greater progress in evolution towards a real civilization than it has made in the past three.

(FMA,*MSI*)

Fundamental concepts of the Alexander Technique

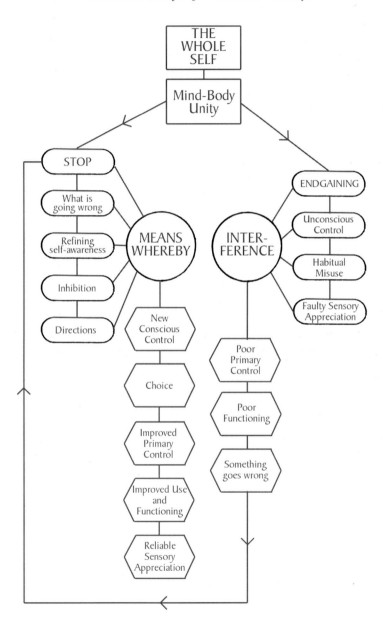

PART TWO

DEVELOPMENTS

MAKING THE TECHNIQUE YOUR OWN

There is a time in the study of all great systems and theories when the student understands the ideas, but experiences them as external to herself; and then there is a time when one internalizes the ideas and principles. They become absorbed into the psyche, a part of one's everyday understanding. When this happens the system begins to grow and expand, as the student applies it to other areas of life.

The Alexander Technique can offer a foundation for all human activity. It can underlie everything we do, every decision we make and every activity we enter into. Alternatively, it can have a fairly limited area of application; many people only apply it to bodily use and movement.

This foundation is based upon a set of principles which together produce an effective method, or means whereby we can create the changes we want to make in our lives, and so we can live our lives in the way we want to, operating from choice and conscious awareness, rather than from habit and subconscious drives. And we can apply these principles to many different areas of life, such as our working life, our personal and emotional life, our mental attitudes in general, and our spiritual understanding.

The same theory can be understood and explained in a myriad of different ways, because it interacts with the life of the person who has adopted it, developing its own particular slant in relation to that person. It is rather like the way a kaleidoscope works: the number of pieces remains constant but the picture changes every time it is moved. A new angle, a new perspective creates a uniquely different picture with the same fundamental pieces. This application and development of the original ideas is a natural process which keeps the ideas rich and alive.

When Alexander began training teachers of the technique he didn't want anybody to copy him. He himself had learnt very little through conscious imitation and he distrusted it as a genuine learning process. He wanted his teachers to make their own discoveries and work things out for themselves as he had done, so that each teacher would have their own unique approach and way of working with the principles.

In the first part of this book I have laid out the building blocks, the pieces of the kaleidoscope, that make up the Alexander Technique, in the pattern that I have found most helpful for myself and my students. In the second part of the book I have developed these ideas, and introduced others that represent ways in which I have applied the technique according to my own interests.

Alexander was ahead of his time, but necessarily he was also 'of his time'. Many of the subjects I introduce in Part Two of this book were given short shrift by Alexander in his writings. He was concerned with the absolute fundamentals of living, and argued quite correctly that while the use of a person is poor and the sensory appreciation unreliable, then everything else about that person's life will be affected by those malfunctionings;

> *To a certain point I am in sympathy with all workers in either 'physical', 'mental', or 'spiritual' spheres, for I believe that 'there are more things in heaven and earth than are dreamt of in our philosophy', but it has always seemed to me that the first duty of man was and is to understand and develop those potentialities which are well within the sphere of his activities here on earth.* (FMA,CCC)

Alexander seemed to believe that by improving the primary control of a person, by means of inhibition and direction of the use of the self, all emotional and nervous problems would eventually disappear. Unfortunately this encourages a confusion between 'inhibition' as Alexander used the word, and 'inhibition' in the repressive sense that Freud used it. In Chapters 11 and 12, I examine our emotional and mental life within the framework of the Alexander Technique. This is not a critique of Alexander's ideas on these subjects, which I believe were greatly influenced by the cultural habits of his time, but a development of his principles as applied to these subjects.

In Chapters 13 to 16, I explore our energic and psychic nature. Our psychic experiences are by definition a result of altered mental states. Because of Alexander's emphasis upon 'conscious control', he was very critical of all altered mental states, such as the trance states brought about by hypnosis. He even criticised creative drawing because it encouraged 'profitless dreaming'. Today, with new understanding of the way the brain functions, and with resulting interest in the value of trance or altered states, scientists and educationalists have recognized the importance of 'profitless dreaming' as a necessary part of balanced mental activity. I am not suggesting that Alexander's concept of 'conscious control' is invalid, but that it needs re-examination in the light of new information.

Only a week before he died, Alexander said to one of his assistant teachers that the work they had begun had only scratched the surface of the egg. He recognised the future potential inherent in his technique, and the need to develop it. I wish to offer the following chapters as a contribution to this potential.

Chapter Eleven

The Emotional Body

Our emotions are such a rich and complex aspect of our being nature that to look in depth at the way they manifest in our minds and bodies would be a book in itself. There are many many different theories of the human psyche, and ways in which we can understand our emotions. It is not my wish to discuss any particular approach or compare different ones, although I do mention one or two different theories to clarify my own point. All these theories involve a belief in inner conflicts, between different aspects of ourselves, some of which operate consciously and some subconsciously. They suggest different ways in which we can work with these conflicts in order to experience life in a richer, more fulfiling way. These conflicts are reflected throughout our bodies, in the musculature, the internal organs, and the nervous system, causing interferences to the free flow of energy through the body. In this chapter I hope to show how the principles of the Alexander Technique can help us to understand and integrate our emotions and inner conflicts, and enrich our self-awareness and growth in these aspects of ourselves.

Cultural Habits

Emotions are a difficult area to explore for many people in Western Society, and especially in England with its tradition of the 'stiff upper lip', symbol for the denial of our emotional experience and expression. It is important to be aware of our 'cultural habits' as well as our individual habits, because there are societies not very far away from England in which emotional life is less repressed. And in England less than two hundred years ago a man would have been thought poorly of if he had what we now call a 'poker face', that is one which betrayed no emotion. This was considered to be a sign of a very poor character, dangerous and untrustworthy. It would be normal for a man to express his grief through tears. Fashions change! Today's 'Big boys don't cry' mentality is a relatively new fashion, or cultural habit.

In Ireland, so close to England, the cultural norm allows for much more emotional expression, and in romantic countries such as Italy and Spain feelings are allowed to flow more freely. Not that these countries are without emotional repression. Twentieth century Western society in general values the mental or intellectual life far higher than the emotional life. Imagine a mother who says of her child 'My child is very intellectual'. There's likely to be a touch of boast or pride in this remark, whereas in the mother who says 'My child is very emotional', one may detect a note of apology or even guilt. It is prestigious to be intellectual, and a nuisance to be emotional. And yet emotions are an absolutely essential part of our being. Just to give this example I had to point out the emotional quality in the voices of the two mothers, one proud, one apologetic. It is impossible to escape from our emotional experience of life, and yet that is often what we pretend to do in the West.

In a similar way it is prestigious to be big and strong, in this society, and rather problematic to be delicate and sensitive. I remember when I began training in the Alexander Technique I would listen with astonishment when teachers praised me for being very sensitive. I had been told I was very sensitive many times in my life, but it had always been meant as a criticism, a part of me I tried to hide or change. I wanted to be tough! Suddenly I was able to see that sensitivity had value and worth. In certain contexts our abilities become liabilities. Because we are not using them creatively they become destructive. This is a common fear with emotions; for many people they are hardly allowed to be experienced, let alone expressed, so they will not allow themselves to let go emotionally because they are afraid they may be overwhelmed by an enormous tidal wave of repressed emotional energy. On the other hand, some people are slaves to their emotions, unable to think or act rationally, and in danger of behaving very destructively. At different times in our lives we have all probably experienced a tendency towards one extreme or the other. 'Falling in love' is one of the few socially acceptable ways of letting the emotional cat out of the repressive bag, and when this occurs people do behave in all sorts of weird and wonderful ways.

Because emotions have been devalued and intellect has been given status in our society, we tend to split off our emotional experience from our thinking. This can happen in two ways. We can suppress our emotions, just 'thinking' we haven't got any, sitting firmly on any rising wave of emotion, and dealing with life in a 'reasonable' or 'rational' way. Or we can 'act out' our emotions, identifying totally with them, and allowing them to rule the 'Self', experiencing extreme emotions over fairly trivial events, and behaving very 'unreasonably'. We either let the thinking rule us, or the emotions rule us, or we jump from one to the other, and create our own individual variations on the two major themes. Just as we all have very individual physical habits

135

and misuses, but with major misuses in common, so do we all have very different emotional habits and patterns, but with common underlying trends.

Many of the problems begin in early childhood, where the 'normal' experience of most children is that they are encouraged to suppress their emotional expression. Put simply, when a child is 'being emotional' (which tends to involve being quite noisy), they are very often either ordered or threatened to stop, or they are encouraged to be 'reasonable' (to think rather than feel). By suppressing the emotional energy it becomes trapped in the body, locked into muscular tensions. And the child learns in time to tell himself to be 'quiet' or 'reasonable', internalizing the demands of his parents, and suppressing the flow of his own emotional experience. Usually when people behave 'over the top' emotionally, they are tapping into a great well of repressed emotional experience which goes back to early childhood and before .* Emotional excess is the other side of the coin to emotional repression. Both are extreme responses, and to a large extent a result of our conditioning.

And so our reasoning and our feelings appear to be in conflict much of the time, and many people are not even aware of this because the feelings have gone underground into the unconscious (that which is not aware), where they will possibly express themselves, through dreams, anxieties, neuroses, depression, or physical illness, which can include the aches and pains, or emotional stress, that bring a lot of people to the Alexander Technique.

However the accepted cultural values of our society are gradually changing as we move into a New Age. The society we live in has become very out of balance because of its emphasis upon a certain set of values, including the upgrading of intellect and physical strength, and the downgrading of emotion and intuition. The nuclear bomb is a gigantic symbol for this, created by a highly sophisticated intellect to manifest the ultimate in physical strength. We've now got so clever we can blow our own world apart. (It is interesting how when things get to extremes like this, their qualities change - the bomb can be seen as a product of high intelligence, and also it can be seen as the grossest stupidity). The creative aspects of strength and intelligence have become destructive as they have become out of balance.

If we lived in a world where emotions were valued highly, then the horror of the holocaust, the emotional content symbolized by the bomb, would be experienced deeply and would be far too powerful and important for the atom or hydrogen bomb

---

*It has been shown that our emotional conditioning begins in the womb, and it can be argued that our emotional patterns were developed long before that in previous incarnations, and that they are reinforced through the early childhood experience.

ever to have been created. People everywhere are recognizing these imbalances. Politically, the peace movement, the feminist movement, the green movement and other grassroots organizations are pushing for change. The intellectual world is confronting these imbalances in philosophy, science and many other disciplines. And the 'human potential' movement or the 'growth' movement, operating at a more personal level, is giving people the opportunity to balance themselves as individuals, and as part of the whole, by paying more attention to emotions, intuitions and sensitivity, bringing these into balance with our thoughts and rational intellect.

• *Looking for Learned Habits* •

I remember reading a delightful story in Nancy Friday's book, *My Mother, My Self*, about a young woman who had just married. One day she was cooking a leg of lamb. Before she put it in the oven she chopped off the bottom of the leg and then put the two pieces side by side in the roasting pan.
'Why do you do that', asked her husband.
'I don't know. That's what my mother always does', she replied.
The husband then asked his mother-in-law why she chopped the bottom off her leg of lamb before cooking it.
'I don't know. That's what my mother always does', replied the mother-in-law.
The grandmother in this story was still alive and there to tell the tale. When the young man asked her why she cut the bottom off her leg of lamb she told him. 'Because my roasting pan is very small, and it won't fit in otherwise'.
We learn so much from our parents, consciously and unconsciously. This is also true of our emotional habits and our personalities. Often we learn an emotional habit by way of unconscious imitation of a parent or sibling, and sometimes the person we learned it from learned it from her parents and so on. And today, it's possible that we have bigger emotional roasting pans than did our forebears, and some of these habits just aren't useful any more.

Write down three qualities you like and three qualities you dislike about your mother.. Do the same for your father, and if you wish for your brothers and sisters, and any other people you were close to when you were a young child.
Now write down three qualities you like and three you dislike about yourself.
Now write down three qualities you like and three you dislike about the people closest to you in your life today (partner, children, friends).

This information can now be examined for patterns. Are there behavioural habits running through from your parents to your children? How many of the qualities you like/dislike in others do you find in yourself?

Emotional Armouring

Because mind, body and emotions are all different expressions of the Self, the whole, they cannot be split off from each other, and our attempts to cut off the emotions will be reflected in the body and the mind. A simple way to describe one of our learning processes is that our emotional experiences in life cause a reflex imprinting on the muscles. So our muscles hold the nervous responses learned by the body through emotional experience. At this level our nervous systems are the same as those of many other animals. A good experience creates a 'positive' imprint on the muscles, and a bad one creates a 'negative' imprint. So there is a reflex mechanism influencing us to recreate the good experiences and avoid the bad ones.

This is fine for animals who don't go in for a lot of logical thinking, but for human animals it can create conflicts. With our capacity for reasoning and consciousness, a conflict between the conscious thought ('I shouldn't be afraid of this') and the unconscious reflex response ('I'm terrified of this') can become a neurosis. It is common when someone has just had a bad experience, like falling off a bike, to suggest that they get on the bike again straight away, in order to avoid a fear of the bike 'setting in' to the body. This is to counteract the muscle imprinting that occurs as a result of that experience. Many people acknowledge that they have irrational fears that make no sense at all. These fears are embedded in the musculature and nervous system, and work through the unconscious mind.

Wilhelm Reich developed this concept with his theory of emotional armouring. He discovered that the negative experiences in life, if they are not allowed to be fully expressed and released, cause the musculature to be defended against fears that are often learned unconsciously from early childhood onwards, and that by working on the body this armouring and imprinting can be released. The release can be experienced as a releasing of the negative emotion, through its experience and expression, or by a re-membering of the initial situation which created the fear and armouring, a returning into conscious awareness, and so a resolution of the conflict between the rational thought and the reflex emotion.

The way we use our bodies, our movements, our postural adjustments, reflect the emotional traumas which have not been released from the past, and also reflect the

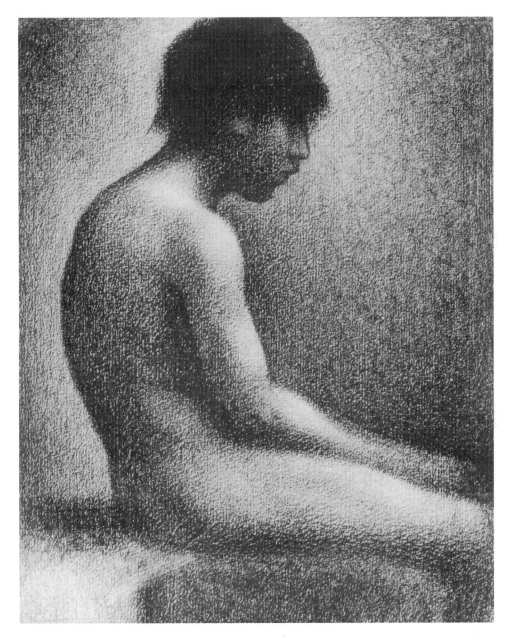

Our muscles hold the nervous responses learned by the body through emotional experience

habitual emotional use learned from our childhood onwards. In my work with drama students it has often been valuable to use this connection between use and emotion. By putting the body in certain positions, or through certain movements, the student is able to contact and recognize associated emotions, and so understand the relationship between physical use and emotional expression in more and more subtle ways. It is the work of the actor and dancer to teach us about ourselves, through the creativity and expressiveness of the body. We can all learn about ourselves in this way, and some psycho-therapists use these techniques to help unravel the emotions held in the body.

• *Contacting the Feelings* •

In this exercise you can work through different movements and positions in order to notice the different feeling qualities that are stimulated. Stay a little time in each moving position until you feel you have explored the emotional experience fully. Describe the physical sensations connected with the emotions.

Example 1. I feel sad and anxious. There's a sensation of heaviness in my tummy, and my heart beat is very noticeable, and I'm getting goose pimples etc.

Example 2. I'm feeling happy. My body is all squirmy and fluid-like. There's a giggly feeling in my throat and jaw etc.

Whenever you have an emotional response, stay with the feeling and if possible allow it to become more intense. If it is unpleasant, allow yourself to contact it for a minute or so and then ask your body for the meaning of the feeling and notice if any images or ideas come through. If you've really got in touch with the meaning you will find there is a shift in the sensations accompanying it, and the emotion may alter. You may find the original feeling was hiding a deeper and quite different one. Explore the new feeling in the same way.

For this exercise and all the following ones please take great care of yourself. These exercises are designed for people who are not suffering from back pain or other acute physical problems.

You need to be in a quiet warm room on a carpeted floor. Lie down on the floor in the prone position, arms down by your sides and with your face turned to one side. Be aware of the emotional feeling of this position, a position you were put down into many times when you were a baby. It may be comforting. It may make you feel restless. Notice how it affects you.

Begin to wriggle around the way a baby would, exploring the movements of your head, arms and legs, and noticing whether this is pleasurable, or uncomfortable or something else.

Staying in this position, make all your body tense. Clench your fists, screw up your face and hold your body as rigid as you can for several seconds, for enough time to notice the changes in your feeling state. Relax and notice the difference. Repeat this.

Now curl up into the foetal position, firstly with your body as relaxed as can be in this position, and then tightening up your body, and then relaxing again, noticing the difference in feeling qualities.

Now lie flat on your back, fully supine, legs stretched out and apart, and arms spread out to your sides. Stay in this position for some time, noticing the sensations and emotions that arise. Curl up into a tight foetal position and then reach out again, noticing the differences.

Lying on your back again, experiment with moving your legs in different ways. Notice the difference when you move the leg smoothly, and then experiment with kicking vigorously. Rest on your back and notice how you are feeling now.

Roll over into crawling and experiment with moving the arms. Once again move them slowly and gracefully, exploring the feeling quality of that, and then make your hand into a fist and make aggressive punching movements.

Still in crawling, arch the back fully, feeling the quality of that movement and position, and then let the back collapse downwards. Now move the back around, up and down, and twisting from side to side, exploring its movement and feeling potential.

Do the same with the head - pull it back. Then let it drop forwards.

Come up into standing. Stand in as balanced a way as you can, giving your Alexander directions, and letting the body be relaxed but not collapsed. Notice the feeling quality of this way of standing.

Now move into a military posture. Pull the head back, and fix it on the neck. Raise the chest up. Pull the tummy in, and the bottom out. Get in touch with the feeling quality of this stance.

Now let the body slump and collapse. Let the head drop, the chest sink, the tummy and pelvis flop outwards. Contact the emotional quality of this position.

Return to the balanced standing position, giving your directions, feeling the chest open but not held up, the neck free, the pelvis free and coming up off the hips. Once again notice the difference in feeling quality.

Experiment with some positions of your own. There are a lot of discoveries to be made, simply by experimenting with different facial expressions.

Notice some of your habitual postures and movements, such as the way you walk. Take time to examine the feeling quality of them.

Emotional Releases During Alexander Work

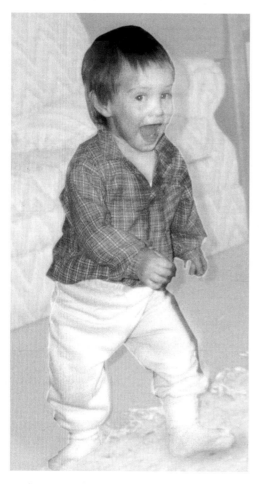

A child expresses joy with his whole body

When a student begins having Alexander lessons, it is quite possible that he will experience emotional releases that are parallel to the physical releases. These may be waves of emotion, such as deep sadness, feelings of vulnerability, or feelings of rage. At other times very positive joyful, or peaceful emotions arise. The student may want to laugh, cry, be angry or just talk about the feelings. Alternatively, sometimes images of past events float into the students mind, often scenes from childhood, that seem to be trapped in the musculature, and as it releases so the memory or image is released. Often a student may feel that he is becoming more alive emotionally, a more generalized experience. After a lesson, students may find themselves much more positive emotionally, because of releases that have occurred during the lesson.

All this is very likely, because of the deep releasing that can occur during hands-on work. These experiences can be most valuable, and are opportunities for insights into oneself, which can greatly assist in developing the refined self-

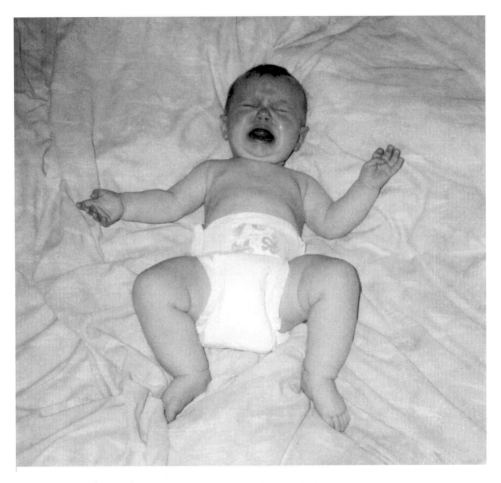

A baby expresses distress freely

awareness that is so necessary to all growth work. Many people habitually ignore this aspect of growth and change, as though emotions are not an acceptable part of the whole self. We need to allow our emotional energy to flow freely and in a well-directed way, just as we learn to allow our physical and mental energy to flow in the best way we can.

Many of my students have worked through emotional changes in their lessons with me. For example, one student of mine found that he stored his anger in his shoulders, and as the shoulders dropped and released, for about two weeks he was subject to increased irritation and anger, although there was nothing 'out there' for him to be angry about. He had stored anger in his shoulders over the years, and it was now discharging. Different parts of the body tend to connect into different emotional energies, but at the same time we are all unique, and create our own particular patterns of muscle imprinting. I remember, during my training, when a teacher worked on my upper chest and rib cage I would often stop the work because I felt very sick and nauseous. One day the teacher suggested I just accept the nauseous feelings and see what happened, and within a few minutes I was sobbing painfully, as my ribs opened and released, and my heart seemed to ache with years of held-in pain and sadness. My way of not contacting my emotional feelings was to hold my breath and feel physically sick.

Another student of mine found, in the course of lessons, that she would contact some very painful emotions and sob quite loudly. She was a person who normally cried very little, and she was quite embarrassed at the expansive expression of emotion that she was capable of. On the rare occasions that she did cry outside of lessons she told me that she did it very quietly and 'politely'. One day she was lying down and I was working on the table with her, and suddenly she remembered the dream she had had the previous night. It had been a very funny dream and she started to tell me about it. I noticed that she was stiffening

This adult is holding on to her distress

144

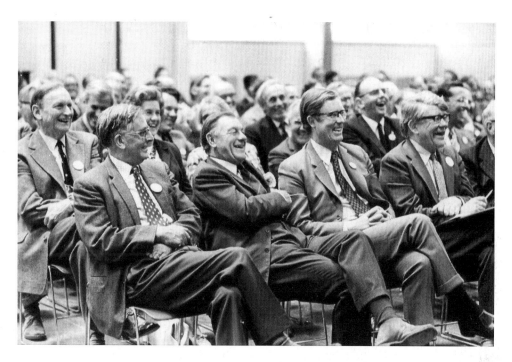

Although laughing, the adults are holding tensions in the body. Notice the hands and legs.

and tightening especially in her tummy, while she talked, so I asked her why this was happening. She said she really felt like roaring with laughter but was embarrassed about doing so. Then she managed to have a good deep belly laugh. We don't only repress negative emotions! How often do we see people laughing really joyously and freely? These positive extremes tend to be repressed just as much as the negative ones. I have found very few people who can laugh without tightening, and yet it is a natural rhythmic release which could happen freely without interfering tensions.

I remember seeing a short film which concentrated on the movements of human beings. It showed speeded-up scenes of children and of adults. It was fascinating to notice how the adult movements were quite clearly the same movements as the children were making, but cut off short, so where a young child would fling out an arm, an adult might move the arm outwards just an inch or two and then halt the movement and hold it within very tight parameters, covering only about 5% of the child's movement. Our civilizing process seems to necessitate this kind of repression at all levels of our being, physically, emotionally, mentally and spiritually.

• Facing Yourself •

For this exercise you will need a full length mirror, a chair, and a notebook and pencil. In your notebook you will need a double page, split into five columns, with the following headings: *Thoughts; Sensations; Emotions; Visual observations; Other:*

This exercise takes quite a long time and is very detailed, so allow plenty of time. Don't rush it. It would be better to work through only a part of the exercise slowly and carefully, than all of it quickly. You can always break the exercise into parts and do it at different times. The importance of this exercise is to give yourself the time and space to discover feelings and thoughts that you may not have known about, so an unhurried approach is essential. Don't endgain!

Sit in front of the mirror and look at yourself for about one minute. Notice what thoughts, sensations and feelings arise as you do this. Stop and note down the things you have noticed, in each of the columns. Notice if you are aware of one aspect of yourself more than another. You may find it difficult to separate thoughts and feelings, so just add that observation to the 'other' column, along with any other observations you find difficult to classify.

Now look again. See if feelings and thoughts are arising that you missed before. What does that person you are looking at convey in that image? What qualities do you communicate through your body image? Accept every single response that surfaces as completely valid. This is how you experience this exercise and so nothing is inappropriate, from embarrassment to irritation to mild terror. Write down your responses once again.

This time pay particular attention to the physical sensations. See if you can observe in the mirror changes that correspond to those sensations. If you feel a lump in the throat, see if you can actually see changes in the throat, perhaps the skin getting blotchy, or the jaw tightening. If you are feeling something in your tummy look at that part of you and see if there is any visible change in that area. Notice what is happening to your breathing. Write down your results.

Now close your eyes and see if you notice sensations better without the visual stimulus. When you have gathered all the information you can, open your eyes, and see if there is anything visible connecting to the sensations you felt (shoulders tightening etc.) Write down your sensations and any visual correlations.

By now you should have a list of physical sensations with some visual correlations. Go through this list and give your attention to the first of these sensations, and see if you can find a thought and feeling that accompanies it. You will possibly feel a connection when you find the related feeling and thought, the sensation will feel a little stronger, or it will dissolve. Write down the correlated feeling and thought for each sensation you noticed.

You may feel there is a more total feeling to which all the individual sensations contribute. See if you can find this. It may help to move your body in the way it wants to go with the sensations. You may want to close in on yourself or shake yourself.

Allow your body to react the way it wants to to this close scrutiny, and see if you can find the accompanying thought or feeling. You may want to laugh or cry or yawn, all forms of emotional discharge. Allow your body to be in charge and respond in the way it will, while your mind observes and notes down your responses.

When you feel you have explored all you can about the sensations arising in your body, and how they connect to visual changes, and to thoughts and feelings arising, make notes on your discoveries.

Once again sit and face yourself in the mirror, and see if there are any new discoveries you can make about your responses. Make notes on these.

• *Bodyscan* •

This exercise is very powerful when done looking into a mirror. As an alternative it can be done lying in semi-supine position, visualizing all the different parts of the body.

Begin scanning your body for thoughts and feelings. Begin with your feet. Look at your feet and observe them carefully; notice the thoughts, emotions and sensations that arise as you do this. The feelings may arise in parts of your body other than your feet. Just keep as aware as you can of everything that is going on.

Now move to your ankles, your calves, your knees, your thighs. Go through the same process with each of these, noting your different responses.

Now give your attention to the pelvic area. We all have taboos about this part of ourselves. Notice how you respond to focusing on your anus and then on your genitals, what sensations, thoughts and emotions are stimulated. Don't worry if your responses seem very inconsistent and contradictory, just allow your being to respond however it will, and accept those responses.

Work your way up through your body, the abdomen, the chest. Watch yourself breathing, and see if you can find the emotional connection with breathing. Is it pleasant, or anxious, or peaceful?

Now give attention to your shoulders, your arms, your elbows, wrists and hands. Now look at your neck, your throat and face. What are your responses to observing your throat? How do you feel about your face? Do you like or dislike it? Which bits do you like, and which do you dislike and why? Note down your thoughts, feelings and sensations as you observe all the details of your face. (The face is such a complex part of ourselves, that you could make this a separate exercise in itself.)

Unreliable Emotional Appreciation

There can be little doubt that the process of reasoning tends to develop more quickly and to reach a higher standard in a person whose attitude to life might be described as calm and collected . . . .

Unduly excited fear reflexes, uncontrolled emotions, prejudices, and fixed habits, are retarding factors in all human development. They need our serious attention, for they are linked up with all psycho-physical processes employed in growth and development on the subconscious plane. (FMA, CCC)

The antagonism between our logical reasoning and our emotions has the potential to be a very rich, creative part of life. The value of emotions is similar to the value of physical sensations, and to our kinaesthetic sense. They put us in touch with our personal inner reality. Our emotional response to a situation is an important aspect of our self-awareness, just as is our physical response, our sensations. It is significant that they are both called feelings.

However just as we suffer from faulty sensory appreciation physically, we suffer from a similar disability emotionally. The devaluation of emotions that is a part of our age and culture means that most people are not sensitively tuned into their emotions, in a subtle moment by moment way. We lack a refined awareness of our emotional experience, either we feel very little, or we over-react to a small stimulus, (in a similar way to which many people feel totally out of touch with their bodies until one day they are experiencing tremendous pain). We also get stuck in emotional habits such as depression, habitual anxiety, or habitual jolliness, and many many more, rather than being finely tuned to the delicate shades of our emotional life.

It is fear of the unreliability of our emotions that makes many people afraid to take them seriously, or to give them the time and space they need to be integrated into the whole self in a constructive way. It is true that the 'calm and collected' person functions better, but a lot of people spend their time pretending to be calm and collected, and covering up a mass of nervous responses with a false persona. This is the equivalent to the person who stands up straight, in a tense fixed way, in order to develop 'good posture'. It adds another layer of tension to the original one.

Interferences to Good Emotional Use

Looking once more at the development of the baby, or the young child, the initial emotional experience is a reaching out for contact, nourishment and pleasure, a simple emotional flow, which becomes distorted if these needs are repeatedly not met. Then the child experiences, and expresses, fear, anger and grief when life is not pleasurable and nourishing any more. These expressions of negative emotion tend to be repressed by authority figures (parents, teachers etc), who teach the child how he 'ought' to behave, how he ought to be quiet rather than noisy, good rather than naughty, right rather than wrong, and so on. The child internalizes and interacts with this teaching in a variety of different ways, and develops a superficial layer of emotional behaviour, which makes up the armouring and defences necessary to adapt to the cultural requirements of the day, and the particular environment of each individual. These adaptations can be very different. One person might be over-anxious to please, while another might be superficially hostile and defensive, and another might find everything extremely boring. At the same time as the layer of superficial emotional activity develops, the primary drives for nourishment and pleasure become distorted and repressed, because they have not been met, as do the 'unacceptable' negative emotions, because they have not been released.

Put simply there are two layers of emotional tension which interfere with our basic emotional drives for contact, nourishment and pleasure. There is a layer of repressed and distorted emotions, trapped in the body over many years. This may seem like the tidal wave of emotion, under the surface, that many people fear. And there is the superficial layer of emotional habits and armouring that we develop in order to cope with everyday reality. If these interferences were removed we would be able to return to that simple state of recognizing and acknowledging our emotional feelings and needs, and experiencing pleasure if they are met and displeasure, which can be experienced, and released, if they are not met.

Alexander students often experience contacting these two layers during their work with the Alexander Technique. In the beginning the effect of the work often seems to neutralize the superficial emotional habits, calming the compulsive tendencies, easing habitual anxiety, and allowing a new tranquillity into the life of the student. But as this defensive layer begins to dissolve, the deeper layer of old repressed pain, fear and anger may begin to surface with the releasing of deeper and deeper muscular tensions. If the student is able to face this 'unacceptable', shadow side of himself then there is the potential for a much deeper level of integration, as old traumas are recognized and released, and the emotional energy is able to flow simply and freely once more. This is the point at which we develop conscious control of our emotions. They are no longer suppressed, and so as they arise, they enter our consciousness, they are accepted and integrated with our reasoning, influencing but not ruling the way we behave, and they are released. At this point our logical reasoning and our emotional experiencing are interacting creatively.

As Alexander said, the problems of our emotional lives must be taken seriously. He recognized the problems, although at that time there was less understanding of how to work with them. Uncontrolled emotions are most unhelpful, but conscious control comes from understanding, accepting and refining our awareness, in the same way as we gain conscious control of the psycho-physical mechanism as a whole. This kind of control is freedom. The primary control of the head, neck and back is the primary freedom of the body. It does not interfere with the energy flowing through the body. As our emotions come into balance they also can flow through our bodies, giving us helpful information about our feeling responses. When we interfere with the emotional flow, we get fixed emotional deadness, or neurotic patterns, on the surface, with a deep well of unexpressed emotion underneath. But the more we can remove the interferences, the more the flow of emotions will be appropriate to the stimulus, and the more trustworthy our emotional responses will become. Just as we must accept the unreliability of our mis-educated kinaesthetic sense, and therefore work to make it more reliable, so we must accept the unreliability of our mis-educated emotions and work to refine them.

• Finding the Faulty Emotional Response •

Although we suffer from faulty emotional responses in a similar way to the way in which we suffer from faulty sensory appreciation, with careful observation we can learn to detect the distorted responses, and distinguish them from straightforward responses. With faulty sensory appreciation, we need the help of a mirror, or another person, preferably an Alexander teacher, to help us refine our kinaesthetic sense. With our emotions it is possible to discover our interferences on our own, although it is still much easier to do it with the help of a friend, or a trained therapist or counsellor.

Learning to observe one's own behaviour with curiosity rather than preconceived ideas is quite a skill to develop. If we can stand back from the picture every so often and consider how we have been behaving, it will become possible in time to distinguish a faulty from a true emotional response. Standing back from the picture is another way of inhibiting, creating a space to look at what is going on.

To begin with it is often easier to create this space at the end of the day. Keep a notebook, and during the evening allow some time to look back over the emotional events of the day. As you refine your awareness of your emotional responses, you will find it easier to 'catch yourself in the act' and observe yourself on a moment to moment basis.

Looking back over the day, did anything upset you? Is it still possible to feel upset about it now? Is your mind still worrying away at the event? If this was a very serious matter then this upset would be appropriate, but if you think the incident was fairly trivial, then you are probably dealing with a faulty emotional response. Something deeper than the actual issue has been stirred up for you, and you now have an opportunity to discover what was going on underneath. Write down your observations.

Did you find yourself getting into a difficult emotional state? There are lots and lots of different kinds. I will give a few examples:

Finding yourself extremely angry over something quite small.
Feeling cold and hostile towards people you normally feel quite close to.
Feeling you are a victim, with no power, and the world has got it in for you.
Wanting to please or impress someone, in an anxious desperate sort of way, needing their approval.
Getting depressed about everything.
Getting anxious about everything.
Needing to feel in control of other people.
Condemning yourself and feeling full of self-hatred, and that you are a dreadful failure.
Being determined to prove yourself right, and justify your behaviour to someone, in an angry obsessive way.

And on, and on, and on. There is no end to the creative variations we find to make ourselves emotionally unsettled and uncomfortable. All these patterns are opportunities for learning, so if they are discovered they can be welcomed and worked with. Write down all your observations. Notice whether your feelings were habitual ones or not. Some emotional states will be very familiar to you, and others less so.

Now remember some of the true emotional responses you made. Think back over the day, and remember emotional experiences that were quite genuine and appropriate. You may have been surprised about this, upset about that, pleased about something else. True emotional responses are positive and negative. They are experienced and then they pass away. They don't leave you feeling uncomfortable for some time afterwards (unless the reasons for them were very serious, and then the deeper and more prolonged response is entirely appropriate and true). Not everything that happens pushes old unconscious emotional triggers that interfere with good emotional use. Write down and acknowledge those moments during the day when your emotional responses seemed appropriate to the situation, and then see what kind of proportion of faulty to true experiences you remembered.

By keeping a record of your emotional experiences, you will soon start noticing you have particular emotional habits. You may like some of your habits, and not like others.

Getting To Know Your Emotional Habits

Just as we can get to know our physical and mental habits of use, and refine our awareness of these, so also with our emotions. Because of many people's tendency to repress the emotions, and not to let them enter into awareness, this process of refining self-awareness may need a lot of careful work. Awareness is the point where thoughts, sensations and emotions meet, but our self-awareness also tends to suffer from misuse and under-development. Our awareness of the outer world has been over-developed and not balanced by an inner awareness of what we are thinking, sensing and feeling.

Our thoughts, our sensations and our emotions are always with us, and always part of what is going on at any moment in our lives. How much we bring those thoughts and feelings into our awareness is up to us. A lot of people prefer to avoid being aware of their emotional life, for fear of the negative emotions that may be stimulated. And that fear is a part of their consciousness, and acts as a block to further development. Moreover it is those negative emotions, locked into the body, that are often the cause of tension patterns, inner conflicts and misuse of the self in the first place. Our negative emotions, even suppressed unconscious ones, are very much at the root of our bad use. Shortening and tightening of certain muscles, pulling down, are all aspects of Reich's muscular armouring. And sometimes the only way to release a muscle is to release the old emotion trapped within it. By ignoring our emotions, we are ignoring the splits and conflicts in our minds and bodies.

Each individual makes her own creative adaptation to the experience of life, and the emotional, physical and mental environment in which she grew up. Inner conflicts develop to deal with outer conflicts, and superficial defences mingle with distorted essences to create the unique and individual person that everyone is. Each person weaves her own web of intricate defences and interacting layers of emotional threads. Eagerness to please may shallowly cover grumbling rage; bravado may paradoxically be hiding great fear; and joviality may be a way of avoiding deep grief. Some people have adapted better than others. Some people have not had to deal with as many difficulties in childhood as others. Some people genuinely do express a more calm and collected manner. For others, to find genuine peacefulness may require a lot of careful and sometimes quite difficult work.

In order to unweave the web, to understand our intricate make-up, and to bring it under our conscious control, it may be necessary to experience and express the powerful and frightening well of emotion of the deeper second layer. It is fear of this that holds many people back from refining the emotional awareness. They have a voice inside them which says, 'I am not the sort of person who behaves like this', and this voice is part of their emotional armouring. There is validity in the fear of releasing a deluge of negative emotion. It has to be done in a safe place, either on one's own or with people who understand and accept the process. Also it is possible to go to the opposite extreme and give too much energy to the emotional experience, stimulating negative emotions repeatedly, until that becomes habitual and out of balance, and therefore in need of inhibition. Ideally we want the stiff upper lip to become still, but in order to do that it may twitch and tremble for a while.

There are many different therapies which help a person develop emotional self-awareness. There are books which teach techniques of self-help, and there are counsellors and psycho-therapists who are trained to help people contact unconscious thoughts and feelings which can rule our behaviour without our knowing why, until we bring them into awareness. Then it becomes possible to discover emotional and mental habits, and find the roots of them. As more awareness develops it becomes possible to understand inner conflicts between thoughts and feelings, and between different conflicting feelings that may occur at the same time. (For example: 'I want to do this, but I ought not to'), Some therapies, such as those following the ideas of Reich, work a great deal through the body, using massage techniques and other methods to release the trapped emotional energy in the muscles. Other therapies such as those following the ideas of Freud and Jung, work more through talking with the client and finding clues through the thoughts expressed by the client. And many therapies use combinations of both.

Each individual must decide and take responsibility for the changes she wants to create. A person who wants to integrate her emotional life more fully will have to choose whether to work on this on her own, or with the help of a counsellor or therapist. And if she chooses to work with a therapist then she has to choose one of the many therapies available, and find a therapist with whom she feels it would be easy and productive to work. I do not wish to recommend one therapy in preference to another, because it is a matter of individual make-up and taste which type of approach is most appropriate. However I do recommend that anybody considering finding any therapist anywhere, for anything, takes two things into account, one is the therapy and the other is the individual therapist. If you feel good about both these then go ahead. If you don't then keep looking.

• Your Body, Your Teacher – Experiencing Your Feelings •

This is a method to help you to look more carefully at one of your emotional responses.*

Choose a situation which, from your observations, you feel you would like to explore more fully. This may be one of your habitual emotional states, or it may be something that triggered off an unusually powerful emotional response in you. It could be something you feel particularly curious about.

Begin by making yourself comfortable and relaxed. I usually start by lying down in semi-supine to do this exercise. Find a space that feels safe and is warm and comfortable. You may want to cover yourself with a blanket. Spend some time becoming quiet and still, so you are in the receptive frame of mind for observing yourself.

Now remember the situation that sparked off the response. Let your mind visualize the details, recalling everything you can about it, until you feel you are beginning to contact the emotional state that it triggered. Now focus on the feelings, both emotional and physical. Describe to yourself how you are feeling, what your body feels like when it is in this state. Imagine you are telling a very compassionate friend all the sensations and emotions involved. Let your body feel them all.

*This exercise, which I devised myself, is very similar to a technique called 'Focusing'. For more information on this read Focusing by Eugene T. Gendlin.

It may help to move into a bodily position that emphasizes the feeling qualities and sensations you are exploring. This may be a curling up into foetal if you are feeling threatened, or a reaching out for some help – whatever feels true to your physical and emotional state. But don't hold this position in a tense way. Relax into it.

If there is a particularly strong sensation, such as a pain in the chest, or over-excitement in the abdomen, it helps to put your hand over that area to encourage the sensation to release, and as it releases to help you understand the meaning of it better. We all have some healing power in our hands, so work with the awareness that you are healing yourself. You may need to move your hand to different parts of your body, as the sensations change.

When you feel you have recreated the experience, pause and be still, and give your attention to what is happening. You now want your body to give you some idea of what this feeling is all about. Ask your self for help, and just watch the ideas and feelings and suggestions that float into your consciousness. Don't intellectualize, or you will get caught up in mental constructions. Stay with the feelings, but with a part of you observing at the same time as feeling.

Ask questions like: Why is this disturbing me? Did I feel like this as a child, and if so when? What is it about this that upsets me?

Watch the responses of your body, as images and ideas float into your consciousness. It is important to work in a gentle way, so that your body can connect into your subconscious, and bring suggestions into your awareness. As each suggestion enters your consciousness, notice how it affects your body. Your body will tell you if the suggestion is appropriate, because the sensations will shift and change in some way.

When the sensations change, you may feel the problem has been released, or you may feel that there are more sensations which are unresolved and need exploring in some way. You may find a lot of tension and anger has released, and you are now feeling very sad and helpless and vulnerable. Then you need to look at the new layer of feelings you have contacted and work with them in the same way.

Sometimes you need to stay with a feeling for a while, especially if it is coming from a deep place inside you that you have not contacted for a long time. Your body will tell you when it wants to change and when it wants to stay with a feeling. At first you may feel you don't know what your body is telling you, but with practice you will be able to tune into your body more and more sensitively, and find it the most reliable of teachers.

Working in this way creates subtle physical and emotional releases in the body, which will leave you feeling much better, as well as helping you to get in touch with some of the underlying causes of the feelings. It also helps to develop trust in your feeling senses, as you bring them more and more into your awareness, and look to them for understanding.

Your Body Your Teacher — Expressing Your Feelings

In the last exercise the emphasis was on experiencing the feelings in the body. Sometimes it is important to express the feeling as well as to experience it. Some people find that by expressing the feeling they contact it more deeply. Other people prefer the gentler experiencing methods of getting in touch with themselves.

There are lots of different ways of expressing emotions. You can write down what you are feeling. You can work with a therapy that encourages expression, such as in psycho-drama. You can get rid of a lot of anger by beating up a cushion, or a punch-bag. (I think a lot of people who play squash have learnt a thing or two!).

The following exercises suggest creative ways of expressing emotions. Working creatively to explore a problem can be highly rewarding. It can release the hold the emotions have upon you, and help you understand your emotional process better as it flows creatively through you, which can be very satisfying. I have emphasized dance because I love dancing, and using the body very creatively, which is a natural development out of working with the Alexander Technique. However it is important after dancing to spend some time resting in the semi-supine position, giving directions and allowing your body to release any unnecessary muscular contractions caused by the dancing.

• *Dance Your Emotions* •

This exercise is the reverse of 'Contacting the Feelings', where you went into a movement or a position to discover emotions connected to it. This time you are going to choose the emotions, and allow your body to express them through movement. One of the best ways of experiencing fully your emotions is to express them creatively; in the process of expressing you may make more discoveries about yourself.

Choose an emotional quality that you have noticed about yourself. It could be one of the qualities you liked or disliked about yourself in 'Looking for learned habits'.

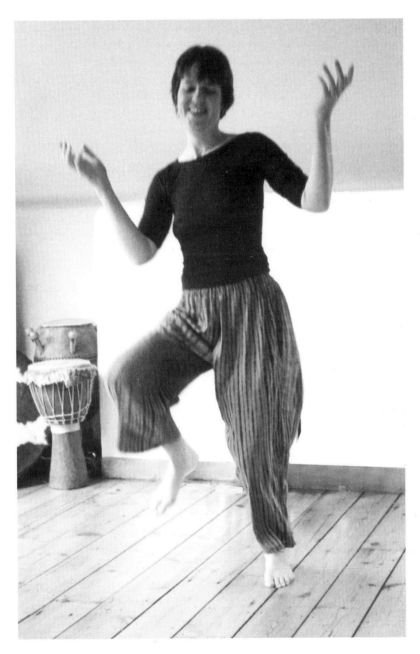

Dance your emotions

For example you may tend to over-react to loud noises, and decide that is the emotional habit to look at. You may have a habit of being terribly polite and ingratiating towards people that you don't really like very much, so you can explore that. You may be very angry about something that has occurred recently and so you can dance out that feeling. Or you may be absolutely delighted about something, so you can dance your joy.

You will need a space in which you can move freely, and where you feel safe and are not going to feel embarrassed because you might be observed.

You can dance to music or not. If you are going to work with music it is important to choose music that is in the appropriate mood, but that will allow you to move out of that mood into others if you need to. Don't let the music dictate your movement. Music that is open to different interpretations is best.

Before you begin to move take notice of the space you have to move in. Place yourself within that space. Feel a part of it. Begin your dance by moving into a stance that suggests the emotional habit or quality you have decided to explore. Allow your body to connect into that feeling and intensify it. Then exaggerate the movement, allowing the feeling and movement together to expand and then to move into something else. Move in accordance with the feeling, not in the way your mind thinks you should move. Don't try to be beautiful, or to 'dance' the way you think dance ought to be. You can dance anything, from ecstasy to ugliness to humour. Try dancing 'Oh, what a fool I must look!', if that's what you are feeling. Just let your emotions and sensations move you into different positions and rhythms. Let your mind observe the process, your feeling centre lead the movement. Imagine you are a young child with no preconceived ideas about how to move and allow the body to make its own discoveries.

Just as you allowed the dance to begin, allow it to end. As you work with an emotional pattern, you will find it either releases or not. If it releases you will find the emotions changing, anger may turn into fear or sadness. Then there will come a point when the emotional quality has worked itself through and there is no emotional charge behind the dance. Then allow the movements to come to an end, finding an ending position in which to conclude your experience. If you have been unable to work through the emotion in movement, then allow the dance to end on the quality of helplessness or frustration that you are left with. Let your body be honest to the emotions involved, however difficult or unsatisfactory they may be. In time that honesty will allow the emotion to surface and be expressed more fully.

After you have danced allow a short time to rest in the semi-supine position, in order to bring your body back into balance. You may feel you have discovered new aspects of your emotional make-up through dancing, or memories and images may have floated into your mind that explained what was happening to you. Or they may not. It is not necessary to have an intellectual understanding of the dancing process. It is therapeutic in itself.

• Find Your Emotions •

You can dance an emotion which you never experience. If you never feel in touch with anger, sadness, fear, or with happiness or peace or some other emotion, then see if you can contact those feelings through movement. Allow your body to teach you its wisdom and experience.

• Dance Your Illness •

Another useful thing to dance is any physical pain you are experiencing, as long as it is not so acute that it would be unwise to dance. You can dance headaches, shoulder pains, tummyaches, and so on. I remember feeling much better when I danced my mouth ulcer. I felt I understood better why I tended to get them, and it healed very quickly.

• Drawing the Feeling •

Just as you can dance a feeling, so can you draw one. Get some wax crayons or felt tip pens, and just as in dancing, allow the emotions to do the drawing. If you're angry you may make some very ugly looking pictures. Great! Whatever you are feeling can be expressed creatively. Notice the changes in your feelings as you work/play in this way.

If you like you can dance your drawing, or draw your dance. Both will help you contact and understand and clear the feelings involved.

Chapter Twelve

The Thinking Body

Thought, I love thought.
But not the jiggling and twisting of already existent ideas
I despise that self-important game.
Thought is the welling up of unknown life into consciousness,
Thought is the testing of statements on the touchstone of the conscience,
Thought is gazing on to the face of life, and reading what can be read,
Thought is not a trick, or an exercise, or a set of dodges,
Thought is a man in his wholeness wholly attending.

D.H. Lawrence

We use the word 'thought' to describe many different aspects of mental activity. Thoughts can be expressed verbally, or through a visual image, or a mathematical formula. Thoughts can be descriptions of the present, memories of the past, or fantasies about the future. So far I have talked about our logical thoughts and our emotions as though they were separate, and as though they were easy to understand in this separate way. But much of the time this is inaccurate, because thoughts and emotions are inseparably bound up together, which is why our attempts to separate them can lead to problems. Thoughts describe reality to us, whereas feelings are our personal experience of reality. Our thoughts are able to observe and recognise our feelings and describe them to us, more or less satisfactorily. (Our lack of refined emotional experience is paralleled by a lack of a refined emotional vocabulary, and so often a person will bring a particular feeling into awareness, but lack the vocabulary to describe it, when they think about it).

One of the attributes of thinking is the ability to make value judgements. When we think, we can think in terms of past, present and future, we can think of what is, and what might be, and so we can make comparisons between alternative situations and decide that one option is better than another. Our ability to choose is based upon our ability to make judgements of relative value. A lot of popular New Age thinking suggests that choosing is a good thing, but judging is a bad one, which is rather confusing. The problem with jettisoning our ability to judge is that we are then in danger of losing our ability to discriminate and to choose, which is no mean baby to throw out with the bath water.

In fact we make judgements all the time. As soon as the statement 'Those are yellow flowers', becomes 'those are beautiful yellow flowers' a statement of fact has become a value judgement. And the difference between the two is that a different emotional quality has entered the arena. Just notice the difference in feeling quality of the following pairs of sentences.

I know Beverley	I like Beverley
He is a football player	He is a poor football player
It is Sunday	Thank goodness it is Sunday.

Sometimes there is a judgement in the sentence when it is spoken, even though it looks purely factual. For example the statement 'I know Beverley' can be said with confidence or uncertainty.

• *Count Your Blessings, and Your Curses* •

Notice how many value judgements you make in the next ten minutes to half an hour. Whenever you think or feel that something is good, bad or indifferent, you are making a judgement. Have a piece of paper beside you and every time you think a judging thought, whether it be positive or negative, mark it on the paper. If you wish you can have two columns, one for negative judgements and one for positive ones. See if you notice how often other people make these kinds of simple judgements too.

• *Speaking with Feeling* •

Choose a nursery rhyme, and say it with different emotional feeling: happy, then sad, then angry.

Now do the same with the Alexander directions. Stand in front of a mirror and say the Alexander directions to your image in the mirror. First say them out loud and then silently. Observe the changes in your body as you say them in different ways.

Free the neck and allow the head to go forwards and up, in such a way that the back lengthens and widens, widening across the upper part of the arms, and sending the knees forwards and away.

Say this in the following ways:

Terribly bored.
Angry and irritated at having to say them.
Looking for approval from a teacher, and terribly anxious to get it right
Calmly and confidently
Try some variation of your own.

Directions and Emotions

Whenever a thought involves a value judgement it carries an emotional quality, and much of our thinking and everyday conversation is brimful of these kinds of thoughts. The amount of thinking we do that is purely factual, or logical is very little, unless we are working as mathematicians or scientists. And even the most factual statement can carry emotion in the way it is expressed. Nevertheless there is a tendency to refuse to acknowledge that this is what we are doing most of the time. People claim they are being scientific and logical, when in fact their argument is based on a lot of very emotive judgements. It is ironic that the theoretical physicists, symbols of objectivity and pure reason, are now the first to accept that their statements are not as objective as they used to believe they were, and the subjective effect of themselves as the observers in their experiments must be taken into account*.

I think the importance of acknowledging the emotional content of our thoughts is absolutely paramount in understanding why our thoughts are so powerful. Thoughts are the means whereby of changing, as Alexander was one of the first to discover, and which biofeedback experiments have subsequently demonstrated scientifically. What gives them their power is the emotional energy behind them.

When you have had an experience of the neck being free and the head moving forwards and up, your neuromuscular system has that positive experience imprinted on it. By thinking the thoughts connected with that experience it is possible for those changes to occur again, or different changes to come about. In other words the directions have a positive emotional content, subtle but very real. Even if a person has no

*For more on this read *The Dancing Wu Li Masters*, Gary Zukav.

direct experience with a teacher of the neck being free, and the spine lengthening, as long as he feels confident about the directions those changes can occur. Alexander sometimes equated 'direction' with 'volition', and the quality of 'wishing' or 'willing' involved in directing shows the importance of the emotional element of the directing thoughts.

If a person connected the verbal directions to a negative emotional experience, the same directions would tend to produce a negative result. Alexander talked a lot about the difficulties of students who became anxious when they gave directions. Similarly, students who are convinced that they are unable to change will prove themselves right. Emotional habits like 'trying hard' and 'wanting to be right' interfere powerfully with the directions. I have seen trainee teachers who have become so utterly bored with the verbal directions that giving them has resulted in a fixing and holding in the head and neck. In order for the directions to work we have to feel good about them, and be confident in them.

We are all very different in our psychological make-up, and for some people the directions given in the same way, day in, day out, can take the form of a beautiful, calming ritualistic experience, and a positive emotional quality then connects to the ritual. For others there is a need for change, new perspectives, new ways of saying the same thing. Once again we need to refine our self-awareness, discover what is working for us, and take responsibility for our own method of working.

• *Semi-Supine Emotional Directions* •

Lie down in a warm carpeted room in the semi-supine position. I am going to give suggestions for thoughts while lying down in this way. Experiment with these suggestions, noting how they affect you.

Think each thought about ten times, observing the effect it has on your body, your emotions, and your mind. Notice if there are physical releases. Notice if your mind starts thinking contradictory thoughts, or your body has contradictory feelings.

When you have experimented with my suggestions, find some thoughts of your own along the same lines. Discover which emotional directions have the most powerful effect on your body.

I am very warm and comfortable lying down in this way.
I am giving my body time and space to release all the physical and emotional stresses of the day.

My mind is full of calm and joyful thoughts.
My eyes look out upon very beautiful things that give me great pleasure.
I hear beautiful sounds all the time. There is peace and silence whenever I want it.
I speak my truth with calmness and confidence. It is easy to be myself,
expressing myself creatively.
Everyone wants to hear what I have got to say.
With every breath the life force enters my body, nourishes me and heals me.
As I breathe in I am fulfiled. As I breathe out, I let go calmly and peacefully.
My shoulders are happy and carefree.
I belong. I am part of the universe. I accept myself totally, just as I am right now.
My arms reach out joyfully to receive all the blessings of life.
I am totally safe. Everybody loves me and thinks I am a wonderful person.
I am a wonderful person.
I am supported by a strong happy back.
I am very successful
My life is deeply satisfying and nourishing.
It is easy to be here, living comfortably on this planet.
My legs are strong and enjoy moving me around.
My legs love being a part of me.
My feet love being in contact with the ground.

I hope you had a lot of fun with this exercise and got an idea of how powerful our emotional directions can be, but if you found it difficult to do because you had a lot of negative reactions to the thoughts, then that's fine. You observed that about yourself which is very useful to know. In the next section we look at that a little more.

Our Feelings Create Our Reality . . .
. . . And Our Thoughts Can Change Our Feelings

'Our thoughts create our reality'. This is one of the fundamental beliefs of New Age philosophy. It is certainly the case that working calmly and confidently with the Alexander directions, in conjunction with inhibition, can bring about fundamental changes in the use of a person.

Alexander was one of the first to recognize the power of thought. And yet it is clear that not all thought is so powerful. I can think, say, shout or sing that today is

Wednesday, and if in fact it is Thursday, nothing I think or voice will alter that brutal fact. If I went on saying it long enough, it would eventually get around to being Wednesday, but it would only last for 24 hours and I think I would be cheating! Thinking is a multifaceted activity, and not all of it can bring about changes. Certain kinds of thinking can, though; they tend to be those thoughts that are verbalized in present tense and can be projected into the future, and that carry some kind of value judgement: thoughts, therefore, that carry an emotional content.

The Alexander directions are a good example. If I tell myself with confidence that my neck is free and my shoulders are widening, although this is a statement in present time, it is in the continuous present, and reaches into the future, allowing the nervous system and musculature to respond to the releasing suggestions.

On the other hand, if I am thinking that my neck aches, my shoulders are tense, and I am feeling awful, the chances are that those thoughts would encourage the situation to deteriorate, and I would either do something about it or gradually feel worse and worse.

Every minute of the day we are thinking little thoughts about ourselves that are dictating to us how we are, and how we are going to be. Usually these thoughts are reflecting our emotional and physical states, be they good or bad. Our thoughts influence our emotions, just as they influence our muscles and our use. Thoughts are the means whereby of change. By thinking in certain ways we can allow change to occur or we can block change. Our thoughts can be creative or destructive, positive or negative, and the way we think, our thought habits, influence the way we are physically and emotionally.

Taking Responsibility

Once we realize the power of our thoughts and emotions, it makes sense to begin taking responsibility for them. Our emotions and our sensations are the means whereby we experience our reality, and our thoughts are the means whereby we confirm or change that reality, depending upon how we use them. Because our thoughts can describe both what is and what might be, we are in a position to influence our emotions and our bodies in whatever direction we choose, if the relationship between our thoughts and emotions is reasonably healthy.

So just as we think of freeing the neck, and that thought allows the physical neck to be freer, so we can think of being happy and fulfiled, and that will give us the opportunity to move into that emotional state.

Affirmations - Emotional Directions

A lot of New Age growth techniques work with the idea of influencing the emotional state by thinking positive thoughts, or affirmations as they are often called. An affirmation is a strong positive statement which can bring about changes in the whole being nature of a person. It is an emotional direction which can counteract a negative habit.

Affirmations can be healing, nourishing, creative, uplifting. They can be thought, spoken, written, sung. Writing a list of affirmations is rather like writing your list to Santa Claus, asking for everything that you want to happen in your life to make you happy. But you write the list as though you've already got it, that is, in the continuous present, because if you write it in the future it will remain in the future and unobtainable. For example:

I am now leading a happy, fulfilled and successful life.
I am now enjoying a deeply nourishing loving relationship.
Everything is working out perfectly for the very best.

If it is possible to change thought habits, so that emotional attitudes to life are fundamentally altered, then it follows that one's experience of life will also be fundamentally altered. In this sense it becomes quite logical to say that 'thought creates reality'. By working with affirmations, instead of living with a set of fearful, suspicious, negative projections about life, we can develop a set of trusting, outward going, confident projections onto the world, and this will certainly create changes in our life experience. Our habitual thoughts, be they good or bad, are our self-fulfiling prophecies about the world, and so by taking responsibility for what we think, we can remove interferences to good emotional use.

By working with our thoughts and our feelings together, we can learn to combine the trusting, open, emotional attitude of the young child with the reasoning and wisdom of the mature adult.

The importance of affirmations is their power to change the physical and emotional state of a person. However, there is a big cautionary note. Because we tend to split off our thoughts from our feelings, it is absolutely essential that if affirmations are to work they do so by connecting and integrating with the emotional life of a person. That involves taking into account the repressed and distorted nature of much of our emotional nature.

A lot of people who are afraid of facing the shadow side of themselves use affirmations as though they can sandblast their way through all the difficult bits, and avoid really recognizing, understanding and integrating them. Then they are simply reinforcing the emphasis on the mental and intellectual side of themselves and this can result in the split between the mental and the emotional life deepening, and the latter going even more unconscious or 'underground'.

People who use affirmations to avoid emotional awareness sometimes have the kind of personality I can only describe as aggressively positive. It is as though the anger they experience at playing this huge trick on themselves has to be used to defend themselves from attack. And so they are saying 'Everything is wonderful, and don't you dare contradict me'.

Another type of person who uses affirmations in this way tends to be very 'spaced out' and out of touch with his body altogether. This very ungrounded person can believe everything is wonderful because he has no connection with his reality, with his emotions and sensations. Affirmations only work if they genuinely change reality, and reality, for us, is experienced through our sensations and our emotions, in a moment by moment way. Unless these change, and unless we are in touch enough with them to know that they are changing, affirmations lead us into a fantasy world which, however beautiful, remains a fantasy from which we will probably come down to earth with a bump.

Endgaining, or Means Whereby

If we use affirmations as a means of tuning sensitively into ourselves, with the object of getting to know ourselves better, rather than using them to endgain, to get results quickly, then we are not in danger of falling into the trap of suppressing our emotions even more, and developing deeper and deeper splits in our being nature. Directions are affirmations. And as Alexander discovered, saying the directions without inhibiting the habitual behaviour is of no value. Nor is giving the directions without careful observation of what is going wrong.

Similarly with affirmations, we need to pause, create space and take time to get in touch with what is really going on, and then let go of what we don't want any more and put the new emotional direction in its place. And in order to 'let go' of a feeling which is no longer useful to us, we need to give time to accept and integrate that feeling, so that the feeling no longer has any charge for us to hold on to. 'Letting go', as the words suggest, cannot be forced. As with many things, affirmations can be helpful or not, depending upon how we use them.

• *Working With Affirmations* •

Affirmations are a way of learning to develop positive thinking habits. But for them to work at a deep level they must connect into our feeling reality in a sensitive way. The following exercises use affirmations as a way of contacting one's deeper feelings, allowing new attitudes to replace the old ones, after the old ones have been recognised and released.

Write down in your notebook two lists: a list of everything that is right with your life, and a list of everything that is wrong with it.

These lists will be used in different ways. The first list allows you to contact your thankfulness about what is working well in your life. It could look something like this:

My health is good.
I'm intelligent.
I like my work.
I enjoy listening to music.
I'm a good cook.
I am very happy with my sexual partner.
I've got some lovely friends.
I like living in this house/town.
I've got no serious money worries.

And so on . . . This list can be encouraged to grow as you think of more and more aspects of your life that you feel good about.

Now for the 'bad' list. Everything that is wrong with your life. Here are some more suggestions:

I don't have enough energy. I'm always tired.
My relationship with my sexual partner is not good.
My work is not satisfying.
I hate my body.
I'm hopeless at coping with money.
My friends don't give me any help.
I get unhappy and depressed very easily.

And so on. These lists can be very long indeed, and that's fine.

• *The Gratitude Process* •

Some people tend to be very conscious of the good things in their lives, and push the bad things under the carpet. Other people focus on their problems and don't notice that many aspects of their lives are problem free and satisfying. Which list did you find easier to write? Were your positive attributes more to the forefront of your mind, or the negative ones? What is your habit, to think the good things, or focus on the problems? If you are problem oriented it will be particularly helpful to you to work with the first list regularly. A person who has an awareness of the good things in her life and an attitude of gratitude at the good things she receives from the universe tends to experience life in a more joyful way.

1) Practise going through your list mentally three or four times a day so you can develop a more balanced awareness of your life.

2) Write the affirmations somewhere where you can look at them regularly.

3) Sit in front of the mirror and tell yourself what is right about your life. Talk to the image in the mirror as though you are a very close friend, using the word 'you' rather than 'I'. (eg. You are intelligent).

Then use the word 'I'. Notice the difference.

When you are working with these affirmations, pay particular attention to your feelings. You may find yourself feeling uncomfortable, sad, irritated, or other emotions that seem inappropriate to the affirmations. This is an important response that needs to be explored. As these affirmations are positive aspects of yourself which you believe are true, this may not occur, and giving the affirmations may simply help you contact positive comfortable feelings about yourself. Whatever your response it's fine. The important thing is to notice it.

If you have a negative feeling, ask yourself why you are feeling bad?

There could be several answers. For example:

I'm not really intelligent, just a smartarse.

All these positive thoughts just make me more aware of the things that are wrong. They depress me.

I hate myself really. This is all bullshit.

Whenever you discover a negative response like this, be grateful that you have observed it. Make a little ritual of thanking the response for coming into your awareness. Then add it to your list of what is wrong. In the following exercises we shall be looking more carefully at these negative responses.

• *The Projects List* •

Take your list of what is wrong with your life, and instead of looking at it in terms of problems, call it a list of projects, a more optimistic approach! Now write a second list, turning every negative statement into its opposite, a positive statement. This is exactly the same as directing the head to go forwards and up, in order to counteract the habit of pulling it backwards and down.

The lists should then look something like this:

I don't have enough energy.	I have all the energy I need.
I am always tired.	I am full of energy.
My relationship with . . . is not good.	My relationship with . . . is wonderful.

And so on. Formulate the positive affirmation, so that only positive terms are used. Don't say 'I am never tired', because the word tired may stimulate a tired response even though there is a negative in front of it. (In the same way one would not give the direction; 'My neck is not tense and fixed', because this could actually lead to tension in the neck.)

When you have written your list of positive affirmations, read through the list and see which of the affirmations really seems to stir up negative responses, ('That's rubbish', etc.) Choose one of these to work with, an aspect of your life that you want to understand better.

Let us use the example 'My relationship with . . . is wonderful'. This time write the list and note down all your responses that surface, good and bad.

For example:

My relationship with . . . is wonderful.	He treats me like a fool.
My relationship with . . . is wonderful.	Our sex life is boring.
My relationship with . . . is wonderful.	He is very generous.
My relationship with . . . is wonderful.	We don't talk to each other enough.

And so on. In this way you are using the affirmation to refine your awareness of the problem. Get to know all your positive and negative thoughts about the problem, and about yourself in relation to it. After you have got as many responses as you can, you may feel you want to explore one response more. Then you can begin a new affirmation around one of the responses, such as 'I have a wonderful sex life', and look into all the responses to that statement. And so you continue to expand your self-awareness.

Affirmations need to be repeated often, to counteract the habitual tendency to think negatively about a subject. And yet the negative responses must be respected and valued. Remember to be grateful for each response you notice; whether you think it is a 'good' one or a 'bad' one it is always a valid aspect of your reality that you have got in touch with.

• *Looking at the Negative Responses* •

These positive and negative thoughts all connect to positive and negative feelings, and it is important to be conscious of the feeling quality of our thoughts. Affirmations can help us to contact our feelings around an issue, if we work with them in that way. In the next exercise I use a combination of affirming positive thoughts, with experiencing feelings which I described in the Exercise called 'Your Body, Your Teacher'.

Suppose you have been working with the affirmation 'I deserve to be happy', and your responses go something like this:

I deserve to be happy	No I don't. Why should I be?
I deserve to be happy	That's stupid.
I deserve to be happy	I don't deserve anything.
I deserve to be happy	I don't deserve to be happy.
I deserve to be happy	I deserve to be miserable. I'm no good.
I deserve to be happy	I'm a mess. I hate myself.

There seems to be an awful lot of resistance to this idea, and it's bringing up a lot of negative feelings. At this point be sure you are in a warm, safe, comfortable space and go through the exercise called 'Experiencing your feelings' (Page 154). Allow those thoughts that you deserve to be miserable, that you are a mess, and so on, to be felt physically in your body. How do you feel? What are the sensations? What feels like an appropriate position for these feelings?

If possible, gently place your hands on parts of your body where the sensations are strongest. You may feel aching in the chest or discomfort in the abdomen. Ask your body to tell you times in the past when you felt like this, perhaps times when you were a very small child. Keep noticing your body's responses, and quietly observing the images, thoughts, and emotions as they rise into your mind, waiting for something that connects to the sensations. You may begin to cry or feel angry or threatened. Allow these responses to arise without interference and be experienced and expressed.

Continue working in this way, until you feel you are getting deeply in touch with yourself, listening to your responses, so that the body gets calmer as it knows it is getting your attention.

Then add the affirmation 'I deserve to be happy'. Direct the thought to where your hands are helping the body to release. You may have your hand on your tummy, which may feel tight.

Feel that you are breathing into that place the words of the affirmation, as part of the healing energy entering that part of your body. Notice the changes that occur, the responses that your body makes, the thoughts that spontaneously surface. The affirmation may make you feel better or it may make you feel worse, until you do release the negative emotion in some way. Think the same affirmation over and over again, always listening for and accepting the response, until it has no more charge. It just feels right.

You might then like to try another affirmation. Maybe in the process of contacting the feeling you thought that the unhappiness came from not feeling good enough for your parents. Then try affirming 'I am good enough', breathing the affirmation into that part of your body that feels most disturbed.

Working meditatively in this way with affirmations, and feeling responses, creates a sensitive integration between the two. Allow the affirmations to contact the related emotions, not to bulldoze their way through them, pretending they don't exist. Then when the negative feelings have been experienced and released, there is a space for the new positive thought to take the place of the old negative one.

Judging, Accepting, and 'Being Judgmental'

Our thoughts carry our emotions, and that is what makes them so powerful, so while it is important to accept the emotional content of our thinking, we need to take responsibility for the quality and degree of emotion involved. Judgement can be very harsh, and can be connected to a very negative repressed emotion. Some people like to distinguish between discrimination and judgement, the former supposedly having no emotional content, and the latter being connected to the negative emotions of anger, resentment, or a quality of blaming. Harsh judgements tend to come in packages like 'You ought not to do that', 'You were wrong to do that', 'That was your fault'. 'Ought' is one of the unacceptable judging words, along with its two ugly siblings 'must' and 'should'.

The reason these words often imply a harsh judging quality is because they are the words we heard as children from the authority figures around us, who were busy trying to socialize us into this society. What we ought to do is usually in contrast with what we want to do. When we are thinking in these ways we are usually being very repressive towards ourselves and others.

Nevertheless I think this distinction is confusing, because it suggests that there is no emotional content in most of our judgements and because it explains an emotional difference by a verbal difference. Discrimination still involves an emotional quality, but it is just not so unpleasant as the heavy blaming or repressive emotional quality that is often called 'being judgmental'.

I think it is important to learn to distinguish between emotional qualities, rather than find the 'right' or 'wrong' words. Sometimes the word 'must' can be used with a very positive emotion attached such as 'I must have a go - it looks great'. There are times when these unacceptable words are quite appropriate and do not carry the negative emotional energies often associated with them, and there are times when judgements are positive and times when they are harsh and negative. It is not differences in terminology, but differences in emotional content that we can learn to be more aware of in our lives.

We need words and thoughts to describe our emotions, but we need to understand the experience of the emotion itself. There is no doubt that if a person is putting out a lot of anger, no matter how well concealed it is verbally, that anger will have an unpleasant effect on those people around him. We probably all know what it's like to be having a conversation about a seemingly unemotional topic and yet for it to be heavy with concealed emotional content.

The tendency to be angry or resentful can be directed outwards and inwards, and often people who judge others harshly also judge themselves even more harshly. This tendency is one of the more destructive emotional habits, and can be very damaging to everyone concerned. More often than not the habit is learned unconsciously in childhood, through the judgements of the parents which then become internalized, as was discussed earlier. People who are very judgmental usually are holding onto a lot of resentment and disappointment from their pasts which they have not accepted and integrated. Blaming and judging others harshly is simply unwise, because we have no idea of other peoples' situations, their inner conflicts and their points of view. Blaming ourselves is equally unwise, because often we are not in touch with our own inner conflicts, and lack a sympathetic understanding of ourselves.

I am not saying we cannot have opinions, or that we cannot have strong negative feelings. But when the two go together in the form of blaming, it usually means there is something much deeper going on than the surface issue. This is the time to pause and examine the situation, and the feelings around them.

We can take responsibility for where we direct our negative emotional energy. We have to make judgements all the time but there is a difference between saying. 'I don't like what you've done' in a tone of voice that indicates that you still care for the person, and saying it with an attitude of blame, condemnation and hatred. Nevertheless if blame, condemnation and hatred are the feelings, I am not suggesting that we suppress them. Quite the opposite, we need to listen to them and be grateful that we are aware of them, because they are an opportunity for learning and growth. Whenever these angry judgmental feelings arise, whether in relation to oneself or to someone else, then it is time to pause and look deeply at what is going on, on the surface and under the surface. If it is possible to inhibit the habitual blaming reaction, but accept the emotions of anger and resentment, then one can open the door to new understanding.

Acceptance

When a person does not have an habitually harsh judgmental attitude, the quality of his responses is one of acceptance. It is possible to feel critical about something but still accept it, ('I do not like this, but I can accept it') whereas it is not possible to attach a harsh angry quality to an attitude of acceptance. When we move to a position of acceptance our view of the world changes dramatically. Everything can be seen as a part of the whole, operating in a way that is totally appropriate to that part. Acceptance puts us in present time, in touch with what is, and not what ought to be. In order to accept we have to be able to let go of the past, and of our expectations of the present and the future. A lot of affirmations involve acceptance, and also forgiveness, as means whereby we can release old unresolved tensions. In order to accept we have to be able to forgive. Forgiving is a way of letting go emotionally.

When Alexander said a student should be pleased to be wrong, he was offering the opportunity to stop being judgmental, and to stop being anxious to be right, and to be pleasantly surprised and curious about the whole process of learning, including being wrong. Unless we enjoy discovering our mistakes, we are not open to learning and improving. An attitude of acceptance is the first prerequisite to the process of refining self-awareness.

It is up to each of us to learn and accept who we are, and how we manifest our reality. Each one of us looks out on the universe but we see it from a different point of view. I can never see things exactly from your point of view and you can never see them exactly from mine, although sometimes we may get close enough for things to look pretty similar. Inside each one of us too there is a universe to discover and explore. There are always bits and pieces in the universe that we don't really like and would rather not see, but if we can learn to accept the whole of us inside, it may affect what we create outside of ourselves. Perhaps if everyone could accept and integrate their inner negativity, we would no longer need to create huge external negativities outside of ourselves. Whenever we blame the world out there for what is not acceptable, and don't see it inside ourselves as well, then we have to project all that negativity into monstrous creations of anger and hatred, like the nuclear bomb.

• Finding Your Judges and Your Baby Rabbit •

We all have our own individual sub-personalities that judge our behaviour, voices inside our heads which nag us, tell us off, sneer and jeer at us. When you are having an intelligent conversation a little inner voice says 'What a fool you are making of yourself. Stop trying to be clever', or when facing a challenge another little voice groans, You'll never do it. You're hopeless'. And on it goes. Every time you take a risk, act creatively, reach out for something you want, the doubting judgmental little voices niggle away, in the background if you're lucky, in the foreground, if you're not.

This is an exercise which may help you discover some of your inner judges, and by getting to know them, accept yourself a little more. *

Lie down in semi-supine, with your head on books. You are going to go into a body scan, as described on page 31.
Let your mind wander over your body, observing it, and attending to the sensations and emotions that arise from it. Your commentary may go something like this:

*Some of the ideas in this exercise come from Eloise Ristad's excellent book on music teaching, *A Soprano on her Head*.

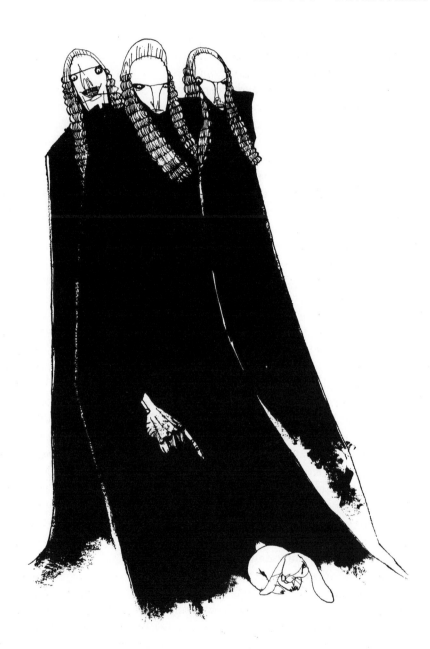

Judges and the baby rabbit

My head feels heavy, and that's OK.
My eyes feel strained and tired, and that's OK.
My shoulders feel tight, and that's OK.
My feet are really enjoying resting against the floor, and that's OK.
My legs are aching, and that's OK.
My abdomen feels relaxed, and that's OK.

And so on.

Every time you add 'And that's OK', notice whether a judgmental little voice inside your head jumps out and disagrees with you. Listen to that voice. It may squeal 'No it's not. Your shoulders should be widening'. This is one of your inner judges. When you hear a judging voice like this, see if you can imagine what the being looks like who owns this voice. You may find you recognise him, a parent, a teacher, or some other authority figure from your past. Or he may be an imaginary character. You may find you have several different types of judges in your repertoire, one who scolds, one who sneers, one who condemns.

Try to bring these creatures out into the open so that you can have a good look at them. Imagine that you are very small and your judges are very very big, towering over you, shouting, screaming, nagging and bullying. Let their voices become more and more grotesque and absurd. Feel the weight of their condemnation.

Now as they stand there, look at yourself and discover that you have turned into a baby rabbit, (or if you don't like rabbits, choose another baby animal). Watch this little creature going about it's daily business, munching a bit of cabbage here, digging a hole there. Now look at these judges descending on this beautiful baby rabbit, who means no harm to anyone, crying out their criticisms, nagging and sneering, and see that baby rabbit astonished by the whole pantomime. After all this little creature is simply being itself. It wasn't to know that farmers don't like holes, or cabbage being eaten, or whatever else the judges may be going on about. Give your love and protection to the baby rabbit, and watch it grow and grow and grow, until it turns back into you, as you are now, lying in semi-supine, lovable and totally acceptable.

Now visualize these judges getting smaller and smaller, as you yourself get bigger and bigger, much bigger than your normal size. If they are real figures from your past it also helps to watch them grow younger and younger, until they become quite young children. Let their voices become small, squeaky and ridiculous. When you feel ten times bigger than them, give them an authoritative look and start talking to them.

'What on earth do you think you are doing ordering me around like this? Have you any idea how absurd you look and sound, and how inappropriate your remarks are right now?' Find words of your own to cut these characters down to size.

When the judges don't feel so threatening it may be useful to have a reasonable adult conversation with them. You could say:

'Look, I know that it would be very nice if my shoulders were releasing and widening, but they are not, and that doesn't mean that I'm a no-good flop. It's quite understandable that my shoulders get tight sometimes, and it doesn't help at all to have you lot making me feel bad about it'.

Your judges may tell you that you do need to maintain a critical eye, you can't lose all sense of discrimination, and you can tell them you know all that, and there's a difference between a criticism which is said with love, care and acceptance, and a harsh judgment. See if you can negotiate an easier relationship with these characters. After all, ultimately they are under your jurisdiction! You're in charge. And remember to see yourself as that baby rabbit, or a baby human as you once were, totally innocent, totally acceptable, as you were then and are now.

Returning to you and your body, go once more through your body scan, making the observations, accepting them, and moving on to the directions:

For example: My shoulders are tight, and that's OK, but I'd like it if they began releasing and widening.

And so on.

• Forgiving Yourself •

Forgiveness is the road to acceptance. Forgive yourself for your mistakes, for being hurt, for hurting other people. And forgive other people for the same. Holding on to old painful resentments leaves no room for joyful new experiences. In order to let go of past hurts you may need to contact the painful feelings in ways I have suggested, but that is better than letting them interfere with your present and your future. Forgiveness affirmations can help with this process.

Another way of working on yourself, that is similar to accepting yourself, is forgiving yourself. For example:

My shoulders are really tight, and I totally forgive myself for this. It's completely understandable that my shoulders have become tight and I feel fine about it. I'd also like it if they widened and released.

And so on.

See how you get on with that alternative. See what your judges think of that! And if you seem to be making progress, see what happens if you forgive your judges for being unkind to you, and forgive yourself for letting your judges upset you, and interfere with your growth.

Inhibition - A Difficult Concept For Post-Freudians

In Chapter Seven I described inhibition as primarily a physiological process. Because the popular meaning of inhibition suggests 'repression', it is one of the most difficult aspects of the technique to grasp. Moreover, Alexander's own writings about inhibition are not always consistent, and are best understood as a development of his own thinking on this subject.

For example, in his first book Alexander describes his technique as a way of enabling human beings to move from instinctual and habitual behaviour to consciously controlled behaviour. He defines the subconscious self as that which governs our instinctual or habitual behaviour, and inhibition as a method of suppressing habitual and instinctual reactions, to allow the possibility of a reasoned response to a stimulus. He describes the development of inhibition in our civilizing process in a way that suggests it is a repressive mechanism:

As soon as any act was proscribed and punishment meted out for its performance, or as soon as a reward was consciously sought – though its attainment necessitated realized personal danger – there must have been a deliberate conscious inhibition of natural desires, which in its turn enforced a similar restraint of muscular, physical functioning. As the needs of society widened, this necessity for the daily, hourly inhibition of natural desires increased to a bewildering extent on the prohibitive side. There grew up first 'taboos' then the rough formulation of moral and social law, and on the other hand a desire for larger powers which encouraged qualities of emulation and ambition.

Among the infinite diversity of these influences, natural appetites and modes of gratifying them were ever more and more held in subjection, and the subconscious self or instinct which initiated every action in the lower animal world fell under the subjection of the conscious dominating intellect or will. (FMA, MSI)

This description does suggest that inhibition is a repressive activity, and his theory was criticised on these grounds. Alexander responded to these criticisms in his second book, *Constructive Conscious Control of the Individual*. He certainly did not want to champion suppression, because inhibition used in the way he understood it was a means to increased freedom, both physically, emotionally and mentally.

> *I shall proceed to show that such an objection is the outcome of a total misunderstanding of the fundamental psycho-physical processes concerned with the application of the preventive principles employed in my technique.*

Of inhibition as used in the suppressive sense, and in relation to the education of children, he says:

> 1. *that the process of inhibition involved is employed in connexion with ideas directly associated with the gaining of 'ends', these ideas being the response to a stimulus arising from some primary desire or need, and*
> 2. *– and this is all important – that the stimulus to inhibit this response comes from without, and the process of inhibition is forced upon the pupil. This means that his desire is thwarted in consequence of compliance with a command from an outside authority, and this could account for the disturbed emotional conditions associated with what is known as suppression.*

Of inhibition in the sense in which Alexander himself used it he firstly remarks that it cannot be understood separately from the practical applications of the principles of his technique. This indicates the physiological nature of the inhibitory mechanism as I have described it. He goes on to say:

> *the process of inhibition – that is, **the act of refusing to respond** to the primary desire to gain an 'end' – becomes **the act of responding** (volitionary act) to the conscious reasoned desire to employ the means whereby that 'end' may be gained.*
> *The stimulus to inhibit, therefore, in this case comes from within, and the process of inhibition is not forced upon the pupil. This means that the pupil's desire or desires will be satisfied, not thwarted, and that there will be present desirable emotional and other psycho-physical conditions which do not make for what is known as suppression in any form*
> (FMA, CCC)

What I find unsatisfactory about these explanations is that our subconscious selves are much more subtle and unfathomable than Alexander believed. He reduces the subconscious to that which rules our instinctual, or habitual behaviour;

> . . . *The subconscious . . . is only a synonym for that rigid routine we finally refer to as habit, this rigid routine being the stumbling block to rapid adaptability, to the assimilation of new ideas, to originality. On the other hand, the consciousness is the synonym for mobility of mind, that mobility which the subconscious control checks and impedes, mobility which will obtain for us physical regeneration and a mental outlook that will make possible for us a new and wider enjoyment of those powers which we all possess, but which are so often deliberately stunted or neglected.* (FMA, MSI)

The work of Freud* and others has greatly enlarged our understanding of subconscious processes. It has explained how the commands from an outside authority can be internalized and appear voluntary and how suppression can arise from internal conflicts within the self. In addition we now know that our brain is organized into two hemispheres with totally different and potentially conflicting functions, the left brain being considered to house the type of logical, analytical consciousness that Alexander was so keen to promote, and the right brain functioning in a very different but vitally necessary way†. Some writers see the right brain as identical to the subconscious. All these ideas were embryonic in Alexander's time, as were his own ideas, and he gave his attention to developing his own theory and practice, and it is left for others who follow and have the advantage of an enlarged perspective to build bridges between the various theories and practices handed down to us, just as there is a bridge between the two hemispheres of the cerebral cortex.

Misleading as some of Alexander's early writings on inhibition appear to be, the concept is fundamental to the Alexander technique, and fundamentally different to the concept that Freud termed 'inhibition'. Freud used the term 'inhibition' to mean 'repression', but to Alexander inhibition is the ability not to respond to a stimulus, thereby creating a pause; time to consider the possibilities in any given situation, rather than to be ruled by habit. For students of the Alexander technique 'inhibition' is a psycho-physical experience which they learn through the guiding hands of the teacher, it is not purely a mental concept. And the experience is one of release in the musculature, freedom in movement and calming of the nervous system. It is not an

---

* Although there are many other theorists to which these arguments would relate, Freud was the father of Psychoanalysis and it is in this symbolic role that I refer to him.
† I say more about this in Chapter Fifteen.

experience of distress that accompanies a repressive act. Inhibition is not an act, it is a non-act. In Alexander's words:

> When it is explained to such a pupil that inhibition is the first step in his re-education, that his apprehensive fear that he may be doing wrong and his intense desire to do right are the secrets of his failure he will invariably endeavour to prevent himself from doing anything, by exerting force usually in the opposite direction. And so he creates a second harmful force which, in conjunction with the first, serves only to increase the undue physical tension and to intensify the already exaggerated apprehensive condition. (FMA, MSI)

That second harmful force is repression. The place in the centre where we can pause and do nothing is inhibition. The difference is subtle but enormous.

> Volition and inhibition are invaluable birthrights of the human creature and should be developed equally, as it were, hand in hand.   (FMA, CCC)

Our volition is our drive, and it is our direction. It is the ability to say 'yes' to a stimulus. Our inhibition is our ability to pause, to think, to consider the alternatives. It is our ability to say 'no' to a stimulus. Both are equally important. We can use inhibition precisely when we feel ruled by an unconscious habitual pattern. Working with the emotions, the first part of the process is the careful refining of awareness of our emotional habits, treating them with acceptance, rather than judging them harshly. And in order to do this we use inhibition, simply to stop and look at what is going on, to say 'no' to the habit of judging harshly, blaming, going into some kind of tirade against oneself or others. We can inhibit the habitual response, and yet give attention to the feeling that charged that response and accept that feeling as a valid reality. Learning to accept is learning to inhibit. And yet even as one part of us is accepting that response, another part is aware that emotional responses are often inappropriate, hiding deeper more difficult feelings. Time must be taken to look for the underlying emotional responses, hidden by the superficial behaviour. Once again inhibition creates the space and time for that self-exploration. At each stage of the learning process, inhibition is necessary.

Inhibition is a continuous process that works through our lives moment by moment, just as volition does. Volition gives us the outward direction in which we want to move, and inhibition gives us the inward direction that pulls us back to our centre, allows us to keep in touch with our true direction, and not get pulled off course.

Freud and Alexander meant very different things by 'inhibition'. Every time you pause to look at an emotional pattern, this is inhibition as Alexander meant it. You pause in order to examine it and understand it better. You don't pause in order to repress the emotional response. This is what Freud meant by inhibition. Our emotional patterns are very individual. One person may have an habitual pattern of shouting and screaming and feeling full of rage when something goes wrong, while another might habitually become rigid and clench the jaw, and feel cold and hostile. Freud would see the clenched jaw syndrome as an example of inhibition, but for Alexander this would not be inhibition at all. It would be a perfect example of an habitual response, as would the shouting and screaming, both equally requiring Alexandrian inhibition to stop the persons being ruled by unconscious habits. For Alexander the enemies were unconscious habits, repression being one example of them. And the way to deal with these habits is to find out what they are, by pausing (inhibiting), accepting them as valid, by inhibiting one's harsh judgments about them, and understanding why they arose, (which might require Freud's help). Having released the habitual pattern it is then possible to look at different possible ways of responding which would be chosen consciously, with more understanding of the situation, rather than being the result of unconscious habits.

Using inhibition in this way allows us to become more conscious of the old patterns of the emotional life. If the behaviour is still expressing a deeply felt unconscious need which has not been released or integrated, we will find it more difficult to inhibit the habit. But if we have already used inhibition to look into the roots of the behaviour, release old trapped negative emotion and integrate the deeper understanding of ourselves, then inhibition of the habit becomes easier. Then the habit has less charge behind it. Finding out how easy it is to inhibit emotional habits is a good way of discovering how much work there is to do on them.

There are always many creative alternatives to an habitual behaviour, as long as one is able to use inhibition. If the emotions involved are extreme then inhibiting may feel like repression. But what you are stopping is the habitual behaviour, not the emotional release. You can then work with the emotions in a more conscious and creative way. As one learns to accept and understand oneself better, the emotional responses become less extreme. But this takes time. The psychotherapist helps the emotional releases to occur which in turn affects the mind and the body, just as the Alexander teacher allows the physical releases to occur which in turn affects the mind and the emotions.

Alexander never worked with emotions in the way I have been suggesting in this chapter. His work focused on the physical use of the body in connection with the mental use of inhibiting and directing.

Working in this way certainly affects the emotions, but he never applied the technique to the emotions directly. Nevertheless I think the principles of the Alexander technique do offer a means whereby we can work directly with the emotions, and that this in turn will have a beneficial effect upon our mental and physical use.

• Looking at the Options •

Once you have stopped behaving habitually you have the chance to behave in an entirely different way. Suppose something has upset you. Below are a list of alternative behaviours for you to play with. Experiment with all the different options, and some more of your own. Give marks out of ten for how well an option worked for you. (You are judging the options, not yourself!)

1. To discharge the energy. This may mean yawning, or crying or shouting and screaming. All these can be forms of emotional discharge. If you are wanting to express anger this can be done using a cushion or other safe inanimate object at which you can direct your negative energy. Or it can be done in the presence of a helpful listening friend, if she's happy to play that role for you.

2. To become rigid, clench the jaw, and feel cold and hostile. (Repressing)

3. To really accept the feelings, to see how they manifest in your body, and to allow the feeling quality of the experience to flow, and ask your body for help in understanding the feeling.

4. To free the neck and send the head forwards and up, in such a way that the back lengthens and widens, widening across the upper part of the arms and sending the knees forwards and away. And see what happens.

5. To give permission for the feeling to be as bad as it possibly can be, so dissolving any fear there may be of really experiencing the negative feeling.

6. To express the feeling creatively, through a poem or drawing or through dance, or drama, and see what you can learn from that.

7. To send all the negative energy into a stone, without acting out. Feel the feel-

ings, then transfer them into the stone. Then wash the stone carefully, and send it some love energy.

8. To think, write, say or sing certain positive thoughts or affirmations about yourself, in order to help you understand your mental, emotional and physical states, and possibly allow them to change.

9. To consider what creates and underpins that feeling and behaviour, and decide to discuss it with a friend, a therapist, or a counsellor.

10. To write everything down that you can think of about the experience, the feelings, the memories it evokes, as a way of clearing it out of your system, and learning more about yourself.

11. To run around the block instead, or jump up and down, or sing a song, and use up the energy another way.

12. To do nothing.

13. To do something else.

Working with the Alexander Technique on the Whole Self

Human beings are so rich and complex in the interconnected aspects of themselves that if we want to become more whole, more integrated, less distorted by interferences whose effects we are not aware of and cannot control, we have many ways of choosing how to create the changes we would like. By giving attention to our thoughts we can learn about our bodies and our emotions; by giving attention to our bodies we can learn about our emotions and our thoughts; and by giving attention to our emotions we can learn about our minds and our bodies. Each leads to the other because each is a reflection of the whole self, each is an aspect of the being nature of each individual, inseparable from the whole. We all have different emphases and preferences as to how we want to create changes, and these too can be taken into account.

Jung postulated dual polarities, thinking and feeling, intuiting and sensing. He thought that people tended to have one dominant pole for each axis, and to have one axis more dominant than the other. For example, one person might be very physically-

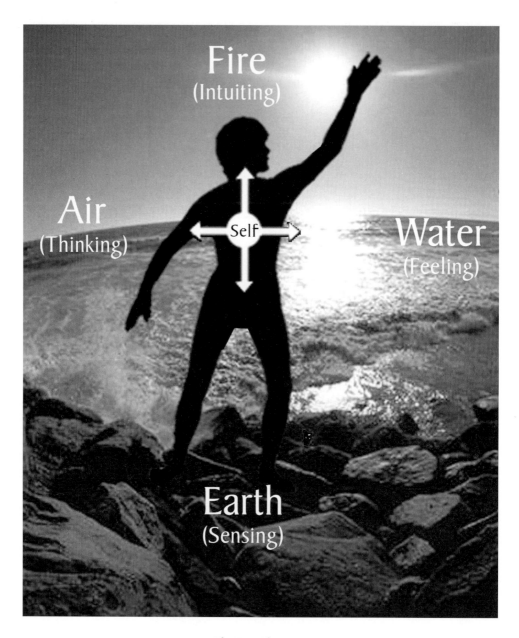

The Four Elements

oriented, based in sensation, and rather weak on intuition, but more comfortable with thinking than with feeling. Another might be very intellectual, out of touch with emotions, and sensations, but also fairly intuitive.

Whether or not this is a good way of summing up differences amongst people it is interesting to look at these four aspects of one's self, and see which of the four aspects one is comfortable with. It may help you to see which ways of working you are suited to, and whether you are neglecting certain aspects of yourself. Each of the aspects is linked to one of the four elements of astrology. To be in balance, all these aspects would be represented equally in a person.

In the symbolism of astrology and other mystical teachings, water is considered the element that symbolizes the emotions, earth represents the physical plane and the body, air symbolizes the intellect, and fire represents our intuition, and our spiritual awareness.

We are living in a period of history which stands astride two ages. The old Piscean age is passing out and the new Aquarian age is moving in. In order to come into balance we have to stand astride several worlds. We have to be able to feel at the same time as thinking, accept at the same time as judging, receive at the same time as giving. We have the opportunity to live in a state of antagonistic flow, balancing all the contradictions that make up our reality. We are all perfect just as we are, and we are all very imperfect, and that's perfect. Instead of opting for one side of the contradiction and letting the other ossify, and be projected onto the outside world, we can sit in the middle of our conflicts and learn to balance the different energies, and in doing so the conflicts become less extreme, our judgements become less harsh, we discover an inner dynamic equilibrium that does not create stillness at the expense of suppression of important parts of us, but finds a harmony in difference. This is peace. It is an inner liveliness, not a static inertia. It is the balance of life and death, light and dark, the goddess and the monster. By owning our own monsters we need not create external monsters. If we accept our internal wars, and let them come to rest, we may not need to create external ones.

Chapter Thirteen

The Dance of Shiva

Energy has mass and mass represents energy.   Einstein, 1905

We have believed for ever so long that matter, stuff is different from energy, just as the body is different from the mind, another form of the same theory. The matter-energy dichotomy goes back at least as far as the Old Testament.   Gary Zukav, 1979

I remember when I first came across Einstein's equation of mass and energy. I was still at school studying pure and applied maths and physics, prior to reading philosophy at University, and so a scientific theory of such tremendous philosophical import filled me with awe and excitement. The world had changed for me, deeply and fundamentally. A table was no longer a solid object, and nor was I! Mass can be transformed into energy and vice-versa.

I also remember my frustration that the objective world did not seem to change so rapidly despite this world shattering news, in fact the only way it did seem to change was literally world shattering, in the form of the atomic bomb, (where massive amounts of energy are released by means of splitting the atom and so transforming its mass). The science fiction films in which people became 'beamed up' satisfied my new understanding of life, but I wanted it to be real, not fiction

After only a few months of training to be a teacher of the Alexander Technique I began to have heightened perceptions. I began to see auras around people and energy flowing, sometimes in the form of colours, and sometimes as though the air was filled with tiny transparent bubbles and streaks. The releasing and changing process that I was going through was freeing me to experience the world in a way that I had blocked. My vision was becoming a reality. The fiction was becoming a fact. Fritjof Capra records a similar experience in the preface to his book, *The Tao of Physics.*

I was sitting by the ocean one late summer afternoon, watching the waves rolling in and feeling the rhythm of my breathing, when I suddenly became aware of my whole environment

as being engaged in a gigantic cosmic dance. Being a physicist, I knew that the sand, rocks, water and air around me were made of vibrating molecules and atoms . . . that the Earth's atmosphere was continually being bombarded by showers of 'cosmic rays', particles of high energy undergoing multiple collisions as they penetrated the air. All this was familiar to me from my research in High Energy Physics . . . but until that moment I had only experienced it through graphs, diagrams and mathematical theories. As I sat on that beach my former experiences came to life; I 'saw' cascades of energy coming down from outer space . . . I 'saw' the atoms of the elements and those of my body participating in this cosmic dance of energy.

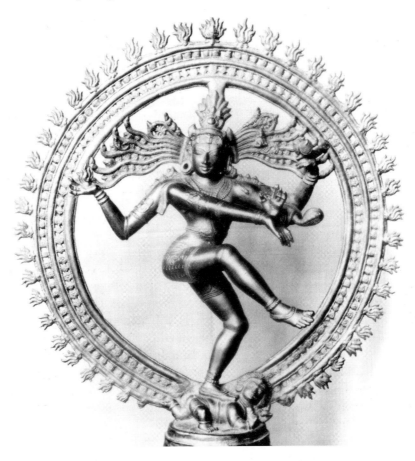

Shiva dancing

When we become aware of what the Hindus call the Dance of Shiva, that the world is an energy dance and that energy and mass are interchangeable participants in that dance, that every particle of matter has an accompanying vibration, that we too are part of that dance, interacting all the time with the environment around us, sending out our own vibrations and receiving others, the idea that we also have a separate self seems contradictory. We live in an age where reality can only be understood in terms of contradictions like these, because we are on the edge of a New Age where reality will take on new meaning for us.

When I began 'seeing things', I became extremely curious and wanted to understand what was happening. It seemed that undoing the muscular and mental tensions, and giving directions in the use of my self, was opening up a kind of clairvoyance (clear-seeing) or psychic awareness. Other teachers and students of the technique have had similar experiences to me, and my curiosity about these experiences, combined with the advice of a psychic who told me I needed to learn the skills of psychic self-protection, led me to study psychic development in England and California, and to develop a synthesis between the Alexander Technique and psychic work.

The first thing I learned about psychic work was that everything was seen in terms of energy. The assumption that mass and energy were interchangeable was fundamental. Physical objects, plants, animals, human beings, the earth and the solar system were all different kinds of energy systems. We give and receive energy from the earth beneath our feet, from the planets and solar system above our heads, and from the atmosphere we live in at the interface of earth and cosmic energy. We also can exchange energy with anything in our environment, other people, or places, or things. In fact it is the collective effect of all the energies that make up the quality of energy in a particular environment, which is why some places feel wonderfully happy and soothing, and others feel unpleasant and disturbing, and so on.

The two disciplines I was learning about seemed to go together very well. Both involved a development of refined self-awareness, and an understanding of the power of mental direction, applied in different ways. I realized that whenever we give anything our attention we give it energy, and the quality of our attention will define the quality of the energy. Scientific experiments with plants have now demonstrated this.* I began to understand the Alexander technique in terms of energy and experimented with 'directions' that involved these energic ideas. I found that by visualizing the Alexander directions as flows of energy I could enhance the quality of the Alexander work I was doing.

I was beginning to make the technique my own.

*For more on this read The Secret Life of Plants, Peter Tompkins and Christopher Bird.

• *Working with Energy Flows* •

Lie in the semi-supine position. Spend about ten minutes observing yourself, getting in touch with what you are feeling and thinking, allowing the muscles to release as you put your body in the position of maximum rest for the spine.

When you feel calm and still in mind and body, bring your attention to your right foot, feel the contact of the sole and heel of the foot with the floor. Now imagine a stream of energy, like white light, entering the body through the right foot. Imagine the light flowing into your foot through the ankles, calves, knees, thighs and hips, into the pelvis and then streaming up the trunk of the body, down the arms, up through the neck into the head and out of the top of the head. As the energy passes through the joints of the body, the ankles, knees, hips and up the vertebrae of the spine, those joints release a little. They become freer, there is more lubrication around the joint. As the light energy flows through the muscles, it releases and lengthens them, so they are coming more into balance. Antagonistic muscles balance each other, both lengthening and releasing.

Now give your attention to your left foot, and go through the same visualization, allowing the light energy to flow throughout the body, not forgetting the arms and hands. If the hands are placed on the abdomen then the energy will flow into the body once more, and up through the trunk of the body into the neck and head.

Now work with both energy flows at the same time. Be aware of the energy flowing through the neck, creating beautiful releases in the muscles and joints of the neck vertebrae. Feel the energy flowing into the head, releasing all the muscles of the face, all the muscles inside the throat and mouth, and freeing the joints of the bones of the skull, so that the fluid moving inside the head flows more freely.

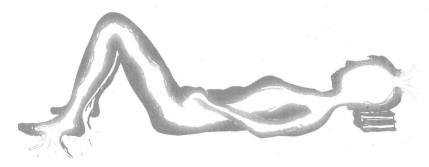

Working with energy flows in the semi-supine

Give your attention to the trunk of your body, allowing the energy flows to release all the tension in the pelvis and abdomen, and in the ribs and shoulders. Imagine the vertebrae of the spine releasing and the spine lengthening, right through to the head. The whole trunk of the body is lengthening and widening as the white light expands and fills it.

Fig. 13.1

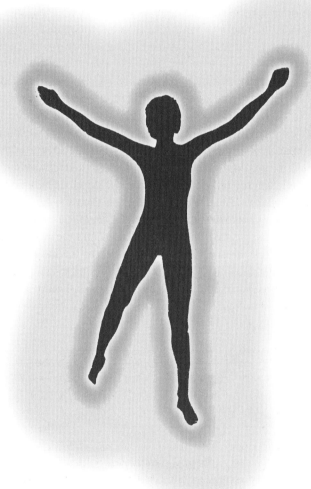

Layers of the Human Aura

Now add another dimension to the flows of energy. In addition to the energy flowing up the centre of the body, visualize it flowing in through the right foot and leg and then crossing the body in a broad band of energy moving to the left shoulder and down the left arm. See the energy, flowing in through the left foot and leg, and crossing over the trunk of the body to the right shoulder and arm. With these diagonal flows the shoulders are encouraged to widen, and the arms and legs are encouraged to be well connected into the back. Feel the flows of energy bringing about the widening and lengthening you want in your body, and the freedom in your neck and other joints that enhances your movement.

The Aura

The Group Field

Pay attention to silence. What is happening when nothing is happening in a group? That is the group field.

People sit in a circle, but it is the climate or the spirit in the centre of the circle, where nothing is happening, that determines the nature of the group field.

Learn to see emptiness. When you enter an empty house, can you feel the mood of the place? It is the same with a vase or a pot; learn to see the emptiness inside, which is the usefulness of it.

People's speech and actions are figural events. They give the group form and content. The silences and empty spaces, on the other hand, reveal the group's essential mood, the context for everything that happens. That is the group field.

John Heider, *The Tao of Leadership*

Every person, every animal, every thing has an aura. Just as the world is surrounded by an atmosphere, so everything in it has its own particular atmosphere, which we call the aura. In effect the aura is the energy field which is created around something. It is the composite of the energies flowing from that object or being, or from a collection of objects and/or beings.

The human aura is very complex and it is affected by the energies of the chakras. These are important energy centres which I will deal with shortly. The aura can be very different from person to person, and even in the same person it changes from moment to moment, day to day and year to year. As we are all changing all the time, so the fluid atmosphere of our energy field changes with us. A healthy aura extends to about one

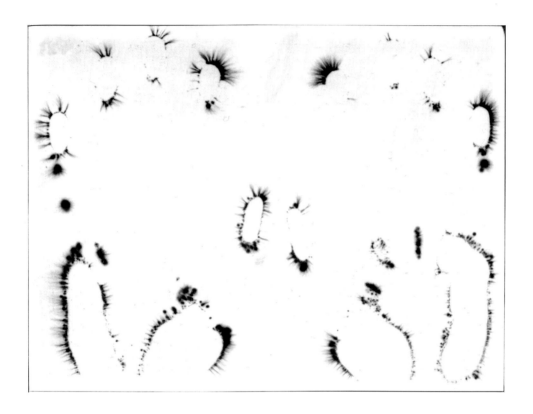

Kirlian photograph of a man's hands, taken when he was very tired

foot all around the body and there are more refined emanations which can be detected several yards away from the body. It is as though we had several different bodies
which exist in different worlds, all interacting and closely interrelated with each other.
There are the physical body, the emotional body, the mental body. Many authorities
suggest seven different layers of the aura, which correspond to the seven major
chakras.

Nowadays, even if you have never seen an aura yourself, it is very easy to see a photograph of an aura. The work of Semyon Kirlian demonstrates photographically the
energy fields around people.

*Subsequent experiments were to reveal that not only subatomic particles but atoms and
molecules as well have associated matter waves . . . Theoretically everything has a wave-*

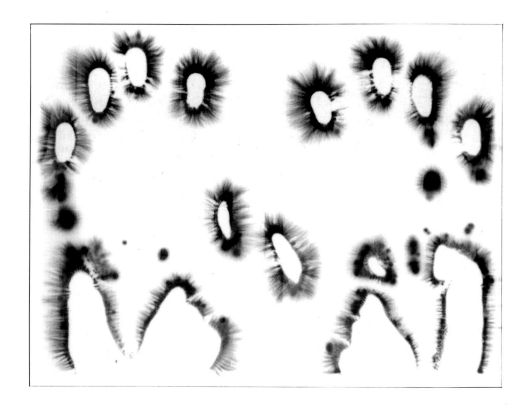

Kirlian photograph of the same man's hands, taken after a holiday when he was refreshed

length – baseballs, automobiles, and even people – although their wavelengths are so small that they are not noticeable.   Gary Zukav, *The Dancing Wu Li Masters*

We are interacting with different energies all the time. The energy of the earth is entering us, the energy from all the different planets and the entire cosmic space above is entering us, and on the earth plane we are in the crossfire of innumerable energy flows from sound, light, radio, electricity and magnetism and many more waves or vibrations that are scientifically understood, and others that are not yet understood so thoroughly, such as the energies from plants, or from our thoughts and emotions. All these energies flow through us and at the same time our own energies flow outwards into the world around us. The invisible world is much greater and more powerful than the visible, but we still tend to limit our sense of reality to what is visible. In the light of modern science it is no longer possible to hold to the old idea that 'seeing is believing'.

When we are in an active mode, moving, singing or talking, even thinking in an active way, or busy 'doing' something, our energy is moving outwards and we are less influenced by energies moving inwards upon us, but when we are in a passive state, daydreaming, listening, watching, waiting, 'being' rather than 'doing', then the energies outside us impinge more noticeably on our minds and bodies.

Many psychically sensitive people are able to see or sense the aura as a band of energy around a person. They may see colours and shapes in the aura. A person skilled in 'reading' the aura can give information about the physical health, the mental, emotional, psychic and spiritual conditions of the person, and even information about the past and the future. We all have these skills to a greater or lesser degree, but they are not developed in our Western culture.

When I was training in the Alexander Technique I was in an ideal situation for developing an awareness of the aura. Throughout the training different people would work with each other, one in the role of student and one as the teacher. Before anybody worked on another person they paused and stood quietly beside the student, inhibiting and working on their own directions. This meant that when I was in the role of student different people would stand by me for a few seconds, without touching me, and I would be able to get a sense of the aura before they actually touched me. What often occurred was that as that person gave directions and those thoughts entered her aura, so I, the student, would find those thoughts working on me before there was any hands-on contact. My head would move forwards and up, my back would lengthen and widen, and I would take a releasing breath with the lovely stimulus. Some had a more powerful auric affect than others, and there would be other qualities I would pick up in that moment of auric interaction, anxiety in some people, a rather blissful healing quality in others, quite a delightful giggly feeling from others, and so on. These qualities changed from day to day, although at the same time most people were 'aurically recognizable'.

Every time you notice an unexpected negative feeling, like anxiety or discomfort or a heavy weariness, in the presence of another person, or alternatively an equally unexpected positive feeling of joy or lightheartedness, as long as you have the sense that it was a bit of surprise, and not something coming from your own state of being, then you are picking up on the emotional energy of another person's aura. The aura has many layers and you can pick up physical symptoms, and thoughts as well as feelings. And you can have the same experience with a place, or a plant, or a stone or anything at all!

Your being receives this complex stimulation all the time. Some people are more sensitive to it than others, and so they may pick up thoughts or feelings of another person, or the quality of a plant, or the feeling of a place. Also some people deal with it better than others, and some (but not all) sensitive people can get quite badly affected by what is going on around and through them, and are unable to control the effect of it upon them. Other people are less influenced by it and are able to operate more consistently despite the differences in energy fields around them. Many people are not aware of their sensitivity and do not understand why they experience mood swings and fatigue or even ill health. I was one of those people, which is why a psychic suggested I study psychic development in order to learn how to deal with the energies around me.

• *Developing an Auric Awareness* •

The following exercises require a free use of the imagination, unless you are able to 'see' auras. If you can't 'see', imagine what it would be like if you could. Imagination and psychic awareness are close relatives. In order to work with either you have to inhibit the interference of the logical, reasonable part of your mind, and allow a different part of your mind to function freely.

Stand quietly inhibiting, and giving your directions. As you get in touch with your kinaesthetic awareness, developing a sense of yourself standing, allow the picture of yourself to include a band of energy about one foot wide, spreading out from your body and encompassing you. Really allow yourself to be aware of how expansive you are when you contact your auric space. Allow that energy around you to be gently flowing outwards from your body, allowing you to expand more and more. Let the aura expand from one foot, to eighteen inches, to two feet and so on. Notice the differences in your body as you expand the aura. Do you feel better as it expands, or do you begin to feel a little unsafe, or do you have some other response? Find out which width of aura feels most comfortable for you. Observe if this is different on different days.

Now begin walking slowly round the room, giving your directions, and being aware of the aura which surrounds you. As you move towards a wall or a piece of furniture notice if you can sense the effect of that object upon your aura, how the aura deals with the object you get close to.

Now move around in any way you wish, exploring movements of the hands and arms, the legs and feet and the whole of the body. Imagine you can see an aura around the hands, the arms, the whole body. How does that auric energy move as you move? What happens if you make a quick arm movement for example? Picture the fluidity of the aura moving around you.

Return to standing again, and pause for a while. Now gently stroke your aura with your hands. Move your hands around your body without touching, as though you are stroking the space around you. See if you can notice the feelings you experience when you are doing this.

It is interesting to experiment with the above exercises using a mirror. Imagine you can see the aura in the mirror around your body. Watch it move as you move. Dance with your aura.

• *Working With Other People* •

If you can explore auras with other people you can get a much better idea of different types of aura. If you have a friend to work with, try the following experiment. Sit in the centre of the room with your eyes closed. Let your friend walk slowly towards you. When you notice her presence tell her what you can feel, what the sensations are, the emotions are, the general quality of the interaction. Let her come even closer to you and continue to give feedback about the auric interaction. Then reverse roles.

When you are with other people, notice what is happening to your aura, and how you feel about their auras. Do they seem to have a very strong expanded aura, or a very gentle receptive one. What does your aura do in response to theirs? People who see themselves as victims contract their auras, and this can make them ill. They don't give themselves enough space. If a person is feeling like a victim it is as though the energy of the world is pressing down on him, so at an energy level he is curling up into as small a space as possible in order to hide from the world. A lot of people tend to merge their auras with whoever they are with, letting the auras flow and blend together. See if you can picture the auras of people you are with, and notice what happens when someone, a friend or a stranger enters your auric space. Begin to notice the subtle changes in feeling when that occurs. Add an awareness of your aura to the general kinaesthetic awareness you are developing with the Alexander Technique.

Chakras

In Eastern philosophy chakra is the name for an energy centre in the body. Chakra is a sanskrit word which means 'wheel', and these energy centres can be seen to turn like wheels, by clairvoyants. There are several hundreds of these centres all over the

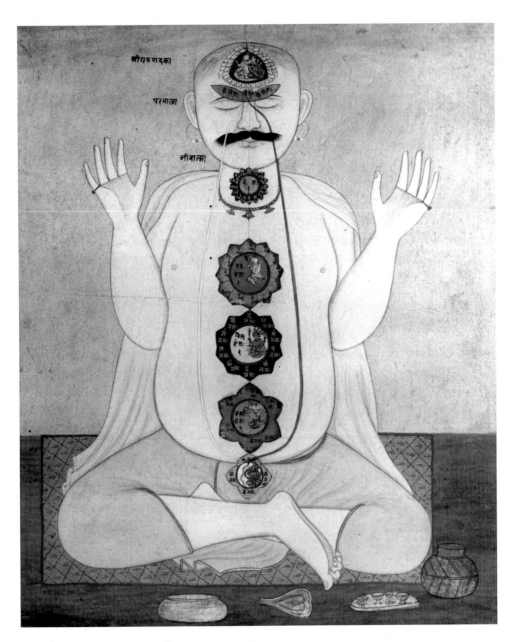

Diagram of the chakras. Kanga state, c.1820

Fig. 13.2

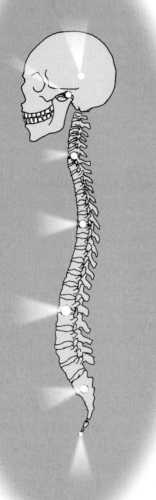

CROWN CHAKRA Pineal gland

EYE CHAKRA
Top of spine / Pituitary gland

THROAT CHAKRA C6/C7

HEART CHAKRA T6/T7

SOLAR PLEXUS CHAKRA L1/L2

SACRAL CHAKRA Sacrum

BASE CHAKRA Coccyx

The Position of the Major Chakras on the Human Spine

body and many acupuncturists believe that they are the same as the acupuncture points in the body. Most of these energy centres are called the minor chakras, and I shall not deal with them here, but there is a group of major chakras, usually considered to be seven in number, (although it can be anything from six to ten according to different philosophies). The major chakras lie up the length of the body, from the base of the spine to the top of the head, and when people talk about the chakras they often mean these major ones. In addition there are important chakras in the hands and the feet.

Quite recently the chakras have been 'discovered' by Western science, using an instrument called an ESM scanner, which works on sound waves. They have also been scientifically treated using electrocrystal therapy. But there is still a lot to learn about the chakras, from a Western scientific point of view, and information coming from different Eastern philosophical sources is sometimes a little conflicting. There are several

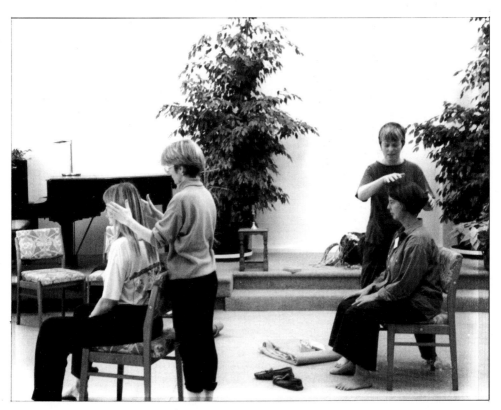

Alexander teachers working on the aura

different systems that explain exactly where each major chakra is and what kind of energy it operates. The fact that there are inconsistencies in these systems points to the need for more research and understanding of these important energy centres.

The system I use, and shall be explaining here, is mainly the one I learnt when pursuing psychic development in California, with small changes and additions which come from my own experience. It is a system relating to Western civilization, and it has proved very reliable in my work over the years. It sees the chakras as operating at different levels of activity. Firstly there is a mundane level in which the different energies of the chakras form the physiological and psychological make-up of a person. So each chakra has a personal psychophysical quality. Secondly, each chakra can operate at a psychic level, which deals with the way we receive energy coming from other people and the outside world, and how we project our own energy psychically. There is also a spiritual level of functioning of the chakras.

In the diagram on page 200 you can see the location of the major chakras. The best way to understand the chakras is to think of them as though they are an energy skeleton for the energy system that is a human being. They organize all the different types of energy in that system. So the chakras and the subtle body, which includes the many layers of the aura, are primary, fundamental parts of us, around which our physical and psychological being is organized.

One level of energy manifestation of the chakras is visible, namely the body. We tend to think of the real world as that which is visible, but this is no longer a workable hypothesis. Light energy makes it possible for us to see a physical world, but it is only a minute part of the energy vibrations of that world. Of the vast electro-magnetic spectrum of energy known to exist, only a minute band is visible light energy. In the same way what makes up a human being is much much more than what is visible, that is, the body.

When we are receiving earth energy, it enters through the feet chakras and travels up the legs to the first chakra at the base of the spine. Energy travels up the centre of the spine through each of the chakras, which are rooted in the spine, and then up into the head and out through the crown of the head. It also travels down the arms, and out through the chakras in the hands.

When we are receiving cosmic energy from above it travels in the opposite direction. The energy enters through the crown chakra and goes down the spine and out through the feet, and also out through arms and hands. In general we give out energy with our hands, but it is also possible to draw energy in through our hands, from the earth and from other sources.

In addition we can draw in or give out energy through the aura, and we are constantly interacting with our environment at this subtle level.

• *Experiencing the Energies of the Chakras* •

The chakras are like wheels which turn clockwise and anticlockwise at different times, possibly dependent on whether they are in an active or passive mode. Experts disagree on exactly which direction is appropriate for which chakra under which circumstances, and I have come across so many variations in my experience I do not wish to put forward any one theory. However it is interesting to experiment and find out how the chakra energy is moving. This can be done by using a pendulum, or by placing the hands in the aura around the chakras. It is best if this exercise can be done with another person, and I will give instructions for this. If you have no-one to work with you can still hold the pendulum or your hand over your own chakras, and this is probably easier done in standing than in lying.

Using the pendulum — The person whose chakras are going to be 'felt' can either stand quite still, or lie down. A pendulum can be made from any object attached to a piece of thread or a lightweight chain, as long as the weight can swing freely.

The person who is using the pendulum holds it between the thumb and forefinger. It should be held lightly with minimum tension in the hand and arm. Using the diagram of the chakras above to locate each chakra, move the pendulum up the centre of the body to where one of the chakras is positioned. Hold the pendulum about six inches away from the body. Now close the eyes and wait. If the pendulum begins to move, allow that to happen. If it doesn't react, move it up and down the spine, trying slightly different positions, until it does begin to move. The important thing is to avoid interfering with the activity of the pendulum, either by making it move, or by stopping it from moving. It is not necessary to close the eyes, but I find it helps to avoid interfering with the pendulum's movements. When the pendulum moves, notice how it is moving, circling or swinging, and in what direction. Write this down as the movement for the chakra, and then move on to another chakra.

Using the hands — This time simply move the hand over the chakras, anything from two inches to a foot away from the body, and notice if you can feel anything. In order to experience the subtle changes of feeling in the hands, you need to be very calm, and in a 'listening' state. Notice changes in sensation in the hand, it may feel hot or cold or tingly or there may be stabs of pain, or other sensations. Experiment with each hand, because sometimes one hand senses energy better than the other.

Chapter Fourteen

The Mundane Level of the Chakras

In the following pages, I give an account of each of the chakras, and its function. I distinguish between a chakra through which the energy flows freely, and a chakra in which there is interference with the natural energy flow. There are different kinds of interference. Difficult experiences in one's life which have not been fully resolved cause trapped energy to get locked in the chakra. This can either block or overcharge the energy flow through the chakra.

For example, an interference can cause attraction or avoidance of our attention. If we get obsessive about food, then there is an interference in the second chakra and it is attracting all our attention. The chakra is overactive in its nourishment seeking. Alternatively an interference may block the energy through the chakra, so we may react by habitually avoiding nourishment, as in the case of people who lose their appetites under stress. Then the chakra becomes underactive. A chakra also may not be functioning normally because the flow of energy from the chakras on either side of it are not balanced. In particular interferences in the energy flow of the lower chakras have a negative effect on the energy flow of the higher chakras.

THE LOWER CENTRES

The Base Chakra   The Root Chakra   The First Chakra

The base chakra is centred on the coccyx, or the base of the spine. The chakra appears to grow out of the spine, so its root is in the coccyx, and a vortex of energy circles out from this point.

Our raw primal energy is stored in the base chakra. It is the chakra of physical, instinctual, animal energy. It deals with essential survival issues, the instinctual drives for food, protection and shelter, the sexual drive at a purely instinctual level. It is about the survival of the self, the 'I'. If a person has problems with the energy flow of this chakra it will tend to manifest in two different ways. She will either be the type of person who takes no risks whatsoever, so afraid is she of not surviving any challenge. Or alternatively she may continually court disaster in order to prove to herself that she can survive. An extremely timid person would be underactive in this chakra, and tend to become ungrounded. An extremely aggressive person would be overactive in this chakra. Both these extremes indicate an obsession with survival issues.

Another way of talking about this chakra is to see it as the chakra by means of which we ground ourselves. We also use the chakras in the feet for this purpose. We are all connected to planet Earth, and this too is an energy system, which we experience as an enormous mass which supports us. Many animals have a tail which can contact the ground, so the base of the spine does extend through the tail to the ground, like an earth link. We receive the earth energy into our bodies through this chakra, either directly or via the feet chakras, and we release unwanted energy formations down into the earth through this chakra in the same way.

When we say a person is very 'ungrounded' or 'unearthed', it means she does not have a strong energy connection with the earth, or a strong sense of physical reality, and often not a strong sense of herself as a physical being. What is actually happening to this person is that the subtle body is splitting away from the physical body, because it doesn't want to experience being in a body. If this happens fully then the person has an 'out of the body' experience. More commonly, when a person feels 'spaced out' it is often a sign that the root chakra is not drawing earth energy into the body very well, so she is becoming ungrounded.

Working as an Alexander teacher I have found that quite often lower back pain and sciatica can be caused by interferences in the root chakra, that is by a person being poorly grounded. Often what occurs is that the person grounds herself through one foot but not through the other, and this creates twists in the pelvis, and the energy flow through the root chakra and the lower back is distorted.

Astral Travel

Some psychics find it very easy to split off the subtle body from the physical body, and they are able to 'astral travel' to anywhere they wish, and return to their physical bodies at will. It is possible that we all astral travel in this way when we are asleep. But for most people being completely 'out of the body' during waking life only occurs at very critical times, such as near death experiences, and for some it is quite frightening and unclear as to whether they will be able to return to the physical body.

The important point is that when this happens we are no longer in contact with earth energy and the root chakra is not functioning normally. Except for those people who have mastered the skill of astral travelling, this usually occurs when the body is in pain, or the person is extremely frightened in some way, and so it is another way of saying the person has survival problems.

• *Grounding Exercise* •

There are many exercises in grounding. I will mention further ones in Chapter 16.

If you are doing this exercise simply as an experiment, I recommend that you give the Alexander directions throughout the exercise, but if you are feeling very spaced out and ungrounded it is better not to give the directions until you feel in contact with the earth again. The direction to send the head forwards and up can be misunderstood and misdirected, leading to more ungrounded-ness, unless well balanced by the thought of the weight going back and down. For this reason I have left the directions out of this exercise.

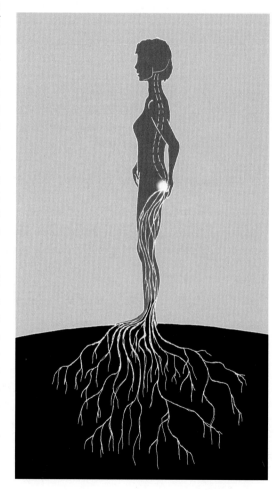

Stand with your feet hip width apart. Be aware of the weight of your body flowing downwards into the earth. Slowly move the weight slightly backwards and forwards on your feet, feeling the effect throughout the body of the weight passing through the front of the feet and then through the heels. Do this about five to ten times, very slowly, giving all your attention to the sensations in your feet as you move, and then come into stillness with slightly more weight on the heels than on the front of the feet. Now move the weight from the left foot to the right, very slowly, once again noticing the changes in your body as your weight shifts. Imagine that below your feet are your roots, like the roots of a tree, extending down into the ground as far as your body extends up above the ground. Place one hand at the front and one hand at the back of your body at the base chakra level so that the energy flowing between your hands energizes the chakra. Continue to sway, forwards, backwards and from side to side, very gently as though you are a tree, thinking always of how your weight is falling downwards through your heels. Now bend your knees a little and continue the swaying movements with your knees bent.

The Sacral Chakra   The Hara   The Second Chakra

The sacral chakra, as its name suggests, is rooted in the sacrum and spirals out from this point. Where the first chakra deals with instinctual and physical energy, the energy of the second chakra is emotional. It gives the emotional context in which a person experiences her reality. It is really about the pleasure principle, the need for deep satisfying nourishment, through good food, loving contact, care and attention, and a sense of belonging. Sexual energy as a form of pleasure, emotional closeness and nourishment is a part of this, and this chakra is often called the sexual chakra, although sexuality at an instinctual level also is active in the root chakra. This chakra also rules the digestive system, and how well we nourish ourselves through the food we take into our bodies.

If this chakra is flowing well, the person is competent at receiving pleasure and nourishment from her life. Usually a person with a strong second chakra is a very happy outward going, kind and generous person. She has learnt very early that in order to receive pleasure you have to be able to give it freely, by being delightful. And because there are no blocks in the energy of this chakra the person will have a healthy digestion, a healthy appetite, and plenty of positive energy, as it is channelled through from the base chakra.

This chakra represents the energy of a young child. If the child is feeling nourished, loved, and included in the family group then she will be full of joy and delight, but if she feels undernourished and neglected then the emotions turn to fear and anger and sadness. The emotions can change quickly from positive to negative, in a young child,

Opposite: *Fig. 14.1* Imagine that below your feet are roots, like the roots of a tree, extending down into the ground.

but if a child experiences habitual neglect, or if she is not allowed to release the negative emotions, through tears or tantrums, then they will interfere with the energy flowing through the chakra. If the chakra becomes overcharged the person may express this through intense emotional moods, or through an obsession for food or for sex. If the chakra is blocked and underactive there might be a holding back of emotional experiencing, or a loss of appetite for food or sex, possibly a rather depressed state. And an obsession in one aspect of the chakra may be covering up for lack of fulfilment of another aspect, such as an obsession for food replacing a need for close sexual contact. The digestive system may be affected, as may the general energy of the person, because she is using the energy of the chakra to either hold down negative emotions, or to overexcite them, and this will interfere with the flow of physical energy of the base chakra.

A lot of the problems I discussed in the earlier chapter 'The Emotional Body', interfere with the energy of the second chakra, in addition to being manifested in the musculature throughout the body. In order to bring this chakra into balance, it is often necessary to move from an underactive chakra to an overactive one, to allow the blocked energy to release. This is another way of saying that for the stiff upper lip to become still, it may need to twitch and tremble for a while. However, we are all unique and the way we interfere with our energy flows is unique, the way we manifest our interferences is unique, and the way we bring ourselves into balance is unique for each one of us. Like the quantum physicists, I can only talk in terms of probabilities.

• Energizing the Second Chakra •

Take a notebook and pen, and find a very comfortable spot, warm and nurturing, and make yourself a hot soothing drink and some tasty morsel to eat, 'a little smackerel of something', as Pooh bear, the archetypical second chakra being, would say, (unless you're very hot and a cool drink would be more satisfying).

Cup your hands over your second chakra, sending it love and healing. Now think of all the things you really enjoy doing. Think of anything that gives you pleasure, nourishment, happiness. Write a list of all the things, activities, experiences, everything you can think of, from horse riding to cups of tea in the garden, anything that gives you pleasure. Imagine some of these wonderful things, as you sip your drink, and savour your smackerel. Read your list every day, and think of one treat, at least, that you can give yourself every day.

A treat a day helps the second chakra play.

The Solar Plexus Chakra The Third Chakra

The third chakra, which is between the navel and the bottom of the rib cage, deals with the development of individual power. It is the largest and most powerful of the chakras. Where the base chakra is focused on survival and the second chakra is focused on pleasure, this chakra is focused on winning, gaining, acquiring, succeeding, being in control of one's life.

When this chakra is flowing well the person has the attitude which is captured by the phrase 'I'm O.K., You're O.K.' He has plenty of self-respect, and confidence in his ability to achieve whatever he sets his mind to. He has a positive ego structure, a sense of dignity about himself, feeling neither superior nor inferior to anyone else.

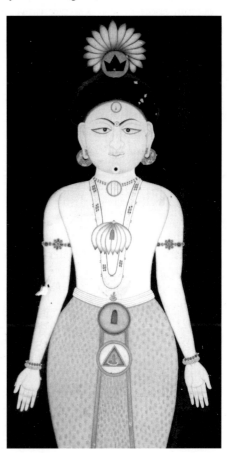

The person with a negative ego structure, who judges himself harshly, the 'I'm not OK, You're OK' person who always feels like a victim, is blocked in this chakra. He has not been able to develop a sense of his own power, and so becomes obsessed with the power out there in the world that he feels subject to. He feels inferior to everyone else, and turns other people into tyrants. The tyrant, or the power crazy person, is overactive in this chakra. This person thinks 'I'm OK. You're not OK', and feels superior to everyone else. Someone who is always out to win, who sees everything including other people in terms of what can be gained from them, or a person who always has to be in control, has interferences with the energy flowing through this chakra.

It is very important to develop a sense of one's own power, and to feel reasonably successful and in control of one's life, without being obsessive about issues of power and control. Whenever you face a

Diagram of the chakras. Rajasthan c.18th.

209

challenge, and do something in order to be able to say that you did it, you are sum-moning the energy of this chakra. When this chakra is flowing well, you are able to deal with conflicts of power in an open and honest way, and you are not afraid of con-fronting difficult situations in order to bring to the surface the issues involved and deal with them constructively.

The positive emotions connected to this chakra are feelings of confidence, dignity and self-respect. Pride, guilt and shame are some of the negative emotions that can block the energy flow, or overactivate it. The victim likes to play on the tyrant's guilt, and the tyrant likes to play on the victim's shame and these types can play these games together endlessly, or until the power issues involved are worked out and the chakra flows freely and easily.

Most people in Western society have blocks and problems in the third chakra because our society is built on the concepts of power and success, and the obsessions of the society naturally become our personal obsessions as well. Also, we often find the needs of the second chakra conflicting with the drive of the third chakra. If you hear yourself thinking that you haven't got time to enjoy yourself, nourish yourself, that there are more important things to do, then you're hearing a conflict between the second and third chakras, and it sounds like the third chakra is winning. The third chakra does a lot of judging. It is usually the part of us that tells us what we 'ought' to be doing, (if we want to be successful, powerful, maintain our self-respect etc.). Allowing harsh judges to become helpful guides is a way of balancing the energy of the third chakra.

• Energizing the Third Chakra •

Here's another list. Write down everything you really like about yourself. 'Judge' yourself as positively as you possibly can, thinking of every positive aspect of your-self, every good thing you've done, every success you can remember in your life, everything you've gained which has enhanced your life, every way in which you feel strong and powerful. Keep adding to the list as you think of more things.

Build up your ego in this way. Then sit in front of the mirror and speak to your-self, saying, 'I am a very wonderful, successful, powerful person. I am in control of my life.' Add to this about ten of the items on your list.

Notice your responses to hearing these self-congratulatory statements. Say them until you can hear that you are saying them with conviction, or until you decide you had better do some deeper work on this issue because it is bringing up a lot of negative feelings.

When you have succeeded in doing this exercise with conviction, think of another person in your life. Don't choose someone close to you, preferably choose someone with whom there might be a certain competitiveness. Now write a similar list about her or him, and say that into the mirror with equal conviction. When you are comfortable about your own power and achievements, and comfortable about the power and achievements of other people (who are not in any way 'in your power'), then the third chakra is coming into balance.

THE HIGHER CENTRES

The Heart Chakra   The Fourth Chakra

Not surprisingly the heart chakra is all about love energy, and how well this flows in our energy system. The love I am talking about is unconditional love, which means simply that their are no conditions to the love. If you feel you love someone when they are doing things to please you, your energy is coming from your second chakra, and is about pleasure. If your love is conditional on status or power in some way it is coming from the emotional energy of the third chakra. If it involves judgement of any kind, it does not belong in the heart chakra. If you love someone *because* they are beautiful, successful or powerful, then that person is energizing your own sense of power and status, which is totally valid, but it is not the unconditional love of the heart chakra. 'I don't love you when you are unkind to me', 'I don't love you when you don't do as I want' – neither of these attitudes belongs in the heart centre. A lot of what passes for love in the world today belongs in the lower chakras, and is a pleasure agreement or a power agreement, or even a survival agreement, which means the love is conditional in some way. A newborn baby usually manages to arouse unconditional love for a time, but the very process of socializing a child involves creating conditions under which the child becomes acceptable, or lovable.

  The unconditional love of the heart chakra is the love of acceptance. It loves a person or a thing for what it is now, unaffected by virtues or vices. It is a wholistic feeling that everything has worth as a part of the whole, that we are all connected and involved with each other, that the world is one great energy system in which everything plays its part. It is love of the 'beingness' of something. It is the love which says simply 'I am', 'You are', and finally, 'We all are', and that is enough. It is a feeling of total affinity with oneself and with the whole of the environment. There are no boundaries, no separateness when the heart chakra is dominating the energy of a person.

The self-concept of a person is held in the heart centre, and of course this is deeply affected by whether one loves oneself or not. Those people who have a sense of their own value, simply because they exist, not because they've managed to survive, or because they experience pleasure, or because they can win, are able to operate from unconditional love, and if they are able to do this for themselves then they are able to love the rest of the world unconditionally. The positive emotion of this chakra is love, the negative emotion is a painful sadness, because most of the time we feel separate and not part of the whole, because we don't accept ourselves and others as we are now.

Traditionally, as a culture, we emphasize the third chakra, but the new age is concerned with developing the energy of the heart chakra. A great deal of the growth movement is involved in the business of trying to get rid of the interferences in this chakra, and in the lower chakras which impede the flow of energy through the heart chakra. In order to allow the heart chakra to flow we must deal with our issues around power, and nourishment, and survival, the issues of the lower centres. For example, if you try to bypass your third chakra stuff, you may end up being a martyr, preaching love energy but having none for yourself, simply imagining you have lots of love for everyone, when in effect you are acting out your need to be a victim, to give away your power in the name of love. Alternatively, you may feel you are loving everyone when in fact the emotion is pride, and you are feeling superior to everyone because you are so 'loving'. It is difficult, in the period in which we live, to separate third and fourth chakra questions, because often our habit is to turn every loving thing we do into an 'ego trip', a sneaky third chakra experience. Every time we make judgements about ourselves, our love, and our loved ones, even if they are positive judgements, we have moved back into the third chakra, out of the accepting energy of the heart chakra. But we have to love and accept even this, as a part of the dilemma of our times. The third chakra often gets into conflicts with the heart chakra. This is the conflict between acceptance and judgement discussed earlier. Of all the chakras, the third chakra likes conflicts most! Through conflicts the third chakra has an opportunity to balance its energy, although often the conflict is just another habit.

When the fourth chakra energy is flowing well, the people in the outside world become real and valid in themselves, whereas in the lower chakras, they are objects of manipulation, in the interests of ego survival, pleasure, or power (ego trip). The boundaries between the self and the rest of the world dissolve when operating from this chakra. Everything becomes part of the whole and valid in itself. Genuine intimacy is possible. A person tends to identify totally with the being nature of another. The energy of the heart chakra is healing energy. The world 'heal' comes from the word 'whole', and as we experience our selves and our world wholistically, so we become healed.

As the central chakra in the body, the heart chakra is the chakra of balance, it balances the energies of the lower chakras through acceptance, and as the energy of the heart chakra develops it allows more energy to flow through the upper chakras. Our chakras develop as we mature. The base chakra is activated through the embryonic period and the first year of life, when the child's main needs are survival needs. During the first year and onwards the second chakra opens as the child needs the emotional reassurance of contact and nourishment. The adolescent experiences the activation of the third chakra during puberty, when normally she gets into many power struggles and conflicts as she asserts her individuality. The heart chakra is the chakra of maturity, when the person goes beyond satisfying needs and is content with everything just the way it is. The upper chakras may then open as that maturity develops.

Of course this is an ideal picture, and most people never remove the interferences in the lower chakras sufficiently to experience a balanced flow in the heart chakra and upper chakras. But most of us have glimmerings of this potential in ourselves. It is what is meant by 'opening the heart centre' which is a popular phrase of the growth movement.* Just as this is the first age to have a wholistic view of the world, so we are now able to develop a wholistic view of ourselves.

• Being Your Self •

Lie down in the semi-supine position. Put one hand at the centre of the chest at the level of the heart and quietly repeat to yourself 'I am'. Do this for at least ten minutes.

The Throat Centre   The Fifth Chakra

This chakra deals with communication. It deals with the way we express ourselves outwardly in the world, and with the way we receive information. It is very creative energy, dealing with song and poetry and all verbal and non-verbal communication. We often forget just how creative it is to communicate. Our voices are very individual, as is our handwriting, and the words we choose to link together, whether we are humorous or serious, to the point, or expansive, all the many permutations in style and content make every communication a creative act quite unique to the person who is making it.

When people talk about opening the heart centre, they mean removing the interferences to its natural easy flow. This is rather different to the psychic skill of 'opening and closing' the chakras at will, which I will explain later.

If the chakra is operating well we are able to communicate what we want to say clearly and in a way that expresses our unique being. We also hear clearly what is said or what is not said, and we perceive verbal and non-verbal communications with similar clarity.

The throat chakra is very much affected by the state of the lower chakras, either consciously or unconsciously. Basically we are expressing all those aspects of ourselves that make up the lower chakras. So if we have problems around receiving nourishment, our voices and what we say will reflect that neediness, whereas if we have resolved those problems it will be easy when necessary to express our need for nourishment in an open and honest way. Similarly if we are power driven this will appear quite clearly in the way we communicate, and if we are comfortable about issues of power, it will be quite easy in a conflict situation to deal openly and powerfully with the issues involved.

If the chakra is not functioning freely, then we are unable to express ourselves clearly. We eat our words, or the words we say are affected by blocks in the lower chakras, so, for example, although we may be trying to express love, people hear messages from the lower chakras that are coming through unconsciously. In a similar way we hear less clearly and are more influenced by our projections, which again will relate to the blocks we have. In other words we hear what we expect to hear. So if we expect someone to be unpleasant, we will interpret the communication as unpleasant. This tends to become a self-fulfilling prophecy, because if we then react as though that person has been unpleasant, the chances are it won't be too long before they really do become unpleasant. This can work in a positive direction too. If you operate as if people love you, you often find that they do! In addition to the blocks in other chakras that affect the throat chakra, the throat chakra can be blocked in itself, if we don't believe we can be creative, or lack confidence in our ability to communicate, to express ourselves, and to listen clearly. It governs our ability to relate to the outside world, both as a giver and as a receiver of information, and so it deals with our ability to relate in general. If the heart chakra is flowing well, and we are relating well in that way, it will enhance our ability to express ourselves and to listen well.

The Brow Chakra   The Third Eye   The Sixth Chakra

The sixth chakra deals with the way we see the world, our intellectual understanding of reality. It is the chakra of logical thought, in that it is the way we deduce how things are in the world, because we have analysed them, pulled them to pieces, and put them in pigeon holes. People who spend a lot of time working with the energy of this chakra are intellectuals, who scrutinize the world to see how it works, theoreticians whether the subject be physics, or the dynamics of human relationships, or the theory of colour. It is the chakra of abstract thinking. If there is an end to be gained through thinking, such as survival, pleasure or power, then this kind of practical thinking operates through the lower chakras.

In addition to deductive thinking, our ability to visualize, to see things in pictures and colours, comes from this chakra.

Our vision of the world is organized from this centre, be it a positive world view or a negative one. So if you are a person who thinks that the world is an evil place, and money is the root of all evil, then you will constantly see the world through the rather grey and drab lenses of that projection, whereas if you believe the world to be abundant and yourself to be fortunate, then you will see the world through 'rose coloured spectacles'. Interferences in the lower chakras will affect your vision. The sixth chakra is the chakra of wisdom and understanding, or lack of it.

Because this chakra holds our vision of reality, it also energizes our sense of purpose in life. If the chakra is flowing well a person has a sense of direction to her life, she feels she is in the right place, 'on the path', whereas if the chakra is blocked a person would either have no sense of purpose, or be a fanatical end-gainer, over-driven and ruthless.

The Crown Chakra   The Seventh Chakra

The crown chakra is the spiritual centre of the body, and it is the centre where the cosmic energy of the universe most powerfully enters the body. It is our link with God, just as the root chakra is our link with the earth. By 'God' I mean an awareness of the whole, and an understanding that is beyond the intellectual pictures we paint with the sixth chakra.

If this chakra is flowing well, we have a sense of knowingness about life, an overview that allows us to be less affected by day to day events. This chakra indicates our autonomy as individuals, the degree of independence that we have in our lives. If we are still very dominated by the opinions of our parents, our cultural background, our friends or our spouses, then this chakra is blocked by those hidden messages that belong to other people. I want to distinguish here between those opinions that you have through choice, (which may or may not be in agreement with your parents and friends etc.) and those which come from habit, and which you have never really examined. These habitual thoughts block the flow through this chakra. If the chakra is completely blocked then the person is totally ruled by the different influences around him during his life, with no personal autonomy. On the other hand, if there are no blocks, then a person is truly connected into the divine flow, is enlightened, is a goddess unto herself, so to speak. Most of us fall somewhere in the middle! This chakra shows the degree of maturity we have attained as a being, in a continuum that moves from slavery to freedom.

The Hand Chakras

The hand chakras deal with our 'giving' energy. They show the way in which our energy system expresses itself out in the world, and in particular how creative we are with our hands. For example an artist will visualize her work through the eye chakra and then express the vision through the chakras in her throat and hands. An artist may be using other chakras as well. If she is feeling very loving then the heart chakra will work through her hands; if she is feeling hurt and angry then the blocked energy of the second chakra will be a part of the work, and it may be that that energy block is released as a result.

The hand chakras also show whether a person's orientation is internal or external, whether their energy goes outwards towards the external world, or inwards towards self-exploration, or a balance between the two.

The Feet Chakras

The feet chakras deal with our 'receiving' energy. We receive the energy of the earth through our feet chakras. If they are blocked then we have problems with grounding, and with receiving in general. All the information about grounding that I have written in relation to the base chakra applies also to the feet chakras.

• Balancing the Energy of the Chakras •

This is a heart chakra meditation which can be done in sitting or standing in addition to lying in semi-supine. In this meditation I shall make use of the colours of the rainbow, which correspond to the seven chakras.

Lie down in semi-supine, and work through your process of self-observation, and then give your directions for lengthening and widening, as laid out earlier in the book. In particular be aware of your back lying against the floor, supporting you. Enjoy the stimulus of the floor upon your back.

Now visualize your spine running through the centre of your body, and connecting to your head.

Bring your attention to your coccyx. Imagine a beautiful red light glowing out from the coccyx. You may see it as a vortex of energy circling out from the coccyx. This is your root chakra. Imagine the red light filling out the whole of your pelvic area and the legs. As is glows and brightens and spreads, say to yourself:

I accept my instinctual nature, that part of me which is purely animal.

Now bring the attention to the sacrum, and see a spiral of orange light moving out from there, filling out the whole of the lower abdomen, see the orange light filling out the space and mingling with the red light of the base chakra. Say to yourself:

I accept my emotional nature, my need for pleasure and nurturing.

Move onto the solar plexus chakra, where the vortex of light is golden yellow. Allow it to fill the whole of your upper abdomen. Say to yourself:

I accept my power, my ability to succeed, my need to have some control over my life.

Let the energy of the heart centre flow giving out a spiral of green light, filling out the chest and shoulders and arms. Say to yourself:

I accept myself totally, exactly as I am now. I am.

Move your attention to the throat centre, the vortex of energy coming from the vertebra (C7) where the neck and shoulders meet, and opening out to where the collar bones meet. Let the blue light fill out the throat, the mouth, jaw and ears. Say to yourself:

I accept the way I express myself in the world. I accept my creative nature.

The brow chakra is between the eyebrows. The colour is the dark blue of indigo, filling out the rest of the head.

I accept my wisdom, my understanding of reality.

Move to the crown of the head where violet light spreads outwards from the crown, and say:

I accept my divinity, my connection with cosmic universal energy.

This exercise can be done as a series of affirmations, rather than statements of acceptance, so you can affirm that you are instinctual, emotionally nourished, powerful, loving and accepting, creative, wise and divine.

You may feel you want to work with one chakra that feels especially blocked. If possible place a hand over the chakra and send it healing (heart) energy. Make the statement of acceptance, or the affirmation about that particular chakra, until you can feel it changing, interferences releasing, and the energy flowing more freely.

Chapter Fifteen

Psychic Level of the Chakras

So far we have dealt with the chakras as they function in our energy system at a mundane level. However, what led me to study these energy centres was that I was experiencing a psychic level of operation, as a result of the Alexander work I was doing. It is not uncommon for a student to find changes of this kind occurring with intensive Alexander work. Releasing the interferences to energy flows means that the psychic level of functioning of the chakras becomes more intense for some people. This may be a very unwanted gift. It is not always desirable to take on another person's thoughts or feelings, or physical pain, and it is important for those people who find they are 'psychically open' to learn how to close down the psychic level of the chakras. Being psychically open can be just another habit, and a very debilitating one.

It is important to distinguish between the two levels of functioning in the chakras. Because while we all function at the mundane level, and we all have the capacity to develop the psychic level (in fact in many people it is something they have suppressed since childhood), it is a skill which develops more naturally and easily in some people than in others, rather in the way that some people are more musically gifted than others. In general, people fall into two categories; those who find it difficult to open up psychically, and those who find it difficult to close down psychically. There are a few fortunate people who are able to control their psychic mechanism easily, without training, so they can operate from choice as to whether it is open or closed. It is a question of one's habitual consciousness. Either one is used to being open or closed psychically. If we can bring our psychic consciousness into our awareness, then it becomes relatively easy to control it, as easy as it is to control any bad habit!

The 'natural psychic' often experiences his skills as a liability rather than an ability because he usually does not know how to control the psychic mechanism, and experiences himself at the mercy of the influences around him. It is because of this, and because I have met many Alexander students who have had difficulties because of their sensitivity, that I wish to explain the psychic level of the chakras, how to be more in control of this level, by learning to open and close the chakras, and develop methods of psychic hygiene and protection. My emphasis in this section is not on showing the reader how to develop psychically, as that would require another book, but on helping the reader to understand the psychic mechanism, and in particular to help those readers who find themselves psychically too open for their own good. In addition the exercises in cleansing and protection are useful and effective for everyone.

Often people talk about chakras being open and closed. This can mean very different things. At a mundane level when a chakra is open, it means the energy is flowing through it in a balanced way. There is no interference to the flow, neither underactivity, nor overactivity. At a mundane level when the chakra is closed then it is underactive. However we have the ability to open and close the psychic level of functioning when we want to. This does not mean that if we close the psychic functioning of the chakra we are also closing its mundane activity. For example it is possible to be very good at expressing oneself, a good communicator, without being constantly open to psychic 'voices' or telepathy.

The mundane and psychic levels of the chakras are interconnected. If a person is blocked in the third chakra, in such a way that he experiences the world from the point of view of a victim, that interpretation of his experience will clearly affect his psychic experience. A paranoid person will be a paranoid psychic, and a trusting person will be a trusting psychic. A lot of psychically sensitive people do have a tendency to be paranoid, because as children they picked up all sorts of information that was then often denied by adults around them, leaving them with a lack of confidence in their perceptions and a lack of trust in other people.

There tends to be a lot of fear and anxiety around psychism. This is partly because it has been suppressed in our society, and in ourselves as children. Also it is worrying because a psychic can have a very powerful influence over others, and those psychics who tend to have a negative view of life can be extremely discouraging in the way they interpret the psychic information. There are two aspects to being psychic. Firstly the psychic receives the information, and secondly he interprets it. Interpretation will be affected by the way the chakras are working at the mundane level. For those who consult psychics, it is important to bear in mind two things. Firstly psychics are fallible. The information they get is not always accurate and sometimes they just get it wrong. Secondly, the way the psychic interprets the information is dependent on the personality of the psychic, and you should assess this in the way you assess any other person in your life. Some psychics are obsessed with the negative and will only be able to pick up information that deals with difficulties and problems. Others are desperately anxious to please and will not receive negative information, or may suppress it, or interpret it in a way that may cloud the issue. Having said this, a good psychic can be a most helpful counsellor, and the skills of psychics are becoming more respected and recognized, in all walks of life, from crime detection to psychotherapy.

The First Chakra (Base)

The base chakra controls our energy supply from the earth. It does not have a psychic function beyond this, but as a supplier of energy this chakra is always open and active, as also is the crown chakra that supplies our energy system with cosmic energy from the universe.

Kundalini Energy

The base chakra does have a further function at a spiritual level, which it would seem important to mention here. It stores the kundalini energy. The Kundalini is an extremely powerful energy resource which can be tapped in times of extreme stress. If you have ever heard stories along the lines of 'Mother, singlehanded, lifts bus off child', then the mother accessed her kundalini energy in those few moments, so powerful was her desire and will to save the child.

The way in which kundalini energy is understood in Eastern mysticism is that if we can raise the kundalini energy through the spine to connect with the crown chakra then we become enlightened. Raising the kundalini can be a dangerous and difficult process if not understood. People have been known to have very painful and terrifying experiences of this when taking drugs. With the right preparation it can be most wonderful and truly enlightening.

The kundalini energy has the power to accelerate the evolutionary development of the nervous system. Our nervous systems work on the basis of muscle imprinting, as I have mentioned before. We have a frightening experience such as falling off a tree, and this fear response becomes imprinted on the musculature, potentially to the extent that every time we are near a large tree we feel afraid. This is the way our neuromuscular system works, just like the rest of the animal kingdom. However as human beings we also have consciousness, and this informs us that there is no reason to be afraid of trees. The conflict between the nervous system and consciousness can develop neuroses. Something frightens us, (such as a spider), which we know consciously is powerless to hurt us. That instinctual imprinted fear can be released when we bring it into line with consciousness, and much of psychotherapy sets out to do this.

The kundalini energy as it rises in the body removes the fear imprinting, and so it brings the nervous system into present time. Every definition of enlightenment involves being in a state without fear, being totally in present time. The rising of kundalini cleanses the muscle imprinting, and if maintained develops a fearless state of being. People who meditate deeply, find old fear and anger states rising up into their consciousness. Meditation, psychotherapy, and the Alexander Technique are all ways of cleansing the nervous system. This is not the same as raising the kundalini energy, which is a powerful physical experience, but it prepares the ground for that transformation to take place if appropriate, whereas the person who

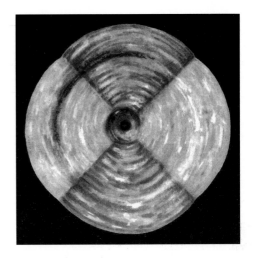

Base chakra as drawn by psychic artist*

experiences the rising unprepared, possibly through the taking of drugs, extreme fasting and other 'forcing' methods usually finds the rising of kundalini an extremely unpleasant and painful experience, as the bright heat and light of the kundalini lights up the old fears and pain of ancient muscle imprinting.

The Second Chakra (Sacral)

Clairsentience, or 'clear feeling' is the psychic function of this chakra and it is the most common form of psychism. Everybody experiences it to a greater or lesser degree. It is the ability to be aware of another person's feelings and physical sensations. We probably all have had the experience of being with someone who is extremely happy or extremely depressed or angry, and finding that we have taken on that person's emotion. Someone who is extremely clairsentient may find that this happens in a shop or a pub, without her even talking to the person near her, and so often not knowing why she has had a sudden mood swing.

*The chakra images in this chapter were drawn by Reverend Edward Warner and can be seen in colour in C.W. Leadbeater's book *The Chakras,* published by Quest Books, Wheaton, Illinois. Notice how the segments of the wheel increase from base to crown chakras.

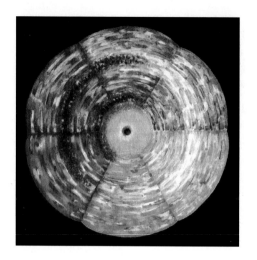

In clairsentience the energy of the other person comes through the aura, and interacts with your aura. A psychically developed person can sense the emotional quality of the other person's aura, but this is different from taking it into her own energy system. If the second chakra is open then you will actually have the feeling, it will seem as though it is yours. You can also pick up symptoms in this chakra, so you may find you have 'caught' someone else's headache or abdominal pain. It is possible to take on another person's illness in this way, either physical or psychological. A lot of illnesses that run in families, such as cancer, can be as a result of the parent's illness being absorbed through the second chakra by the child, although of course dietary and life habits also contribute to these familial tendencies, so it is difficult to prove a primary cause. Heredity plays a part but not as big a part as we tend to suppose. We can absorb the emotional habits of our parents through this chakra, and this can be for better or for worse. In order to be in control of this chakra, the first thing to do is to develop an awareness of your auric experiences, which is another aspect of refining your self-awareness. The exercises on the aura help with this.

The Third Chakra (Solar Plexus)

This chakra moves the energy around the body. Just as it deals with issues of power and control at a mundane level it controls the energy (more or less powerfully) at a psychic level. It is the psychic pump of the body. This affects how we operate at the mundane level. For example if you are feeling very sad, because you are missing the company of someone you love, and you are unable to move out of that sad state although you want to, then you are 'stuck' in the second chakra, experiencing lack of pleasure and nourishment. It may be important to experience those feelings, and you may choose to stay with them. On the other hand you may choose to change your energy state by reading a book which stimulates you mentally, so you are now using the energy of the sixth chakra. Perhaps you may choose to stay with the feelings and work with them in some way, as suggested in the chapter on emotions. Then you will still be using some sixth chakra energy to throw some light on your feelings, and perhaps some heart chakra energy is used to accept your feelings. It is the third chakra that moves the energy around the body, from the second chakra to the sixth chakra, or if you decide to write a poem about it, you will be moving into fifth chakra energy. If you stay sad and miserable when reading, or unable to write a poem, wishing to move out of that state, but not being

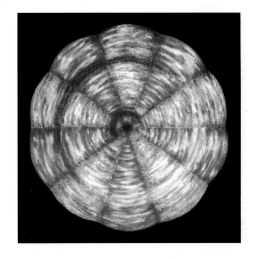

able to, then the third chakra has not succeeded in moving the energy to another centre. The third chakra can also move energy around outside your body. You may wish to send love energy to another person, then the third chakra will move the energy of the heart chakra outwards to that other person. The third chakra also draws energy in from outside and distributes it around the other chakras.

The Fourth Chakra (Heart)

This is the chakra of love energy and at a psychic level the energy is one of total affinity with another. One energically becomes the 'other', whether it is another person or an object. The heart chakra deals with the wholistic experience of life, and so it does not have ego boundaries in the same way as the lower chakras do. A psychic who works from this centre, for a short time 'becomes' the other person, knows them totally, their thoughts, their feelings, their total psychological make-up and physiology. There is a total identification and affinity which is more than the symptom collecting of the second chakra. Most psychics find it difficult to operate from this centre professionally, because they lose their own boundaries and sense of space.

Couples who have lived together for so long that they begin to look alike are usually operating from the heart centre psychically with each other. In time, with this centre, you literally start becoming the other person, because there are no boundaries between you.

Healing energy comes from this centre and is another form of psychic energy. Many

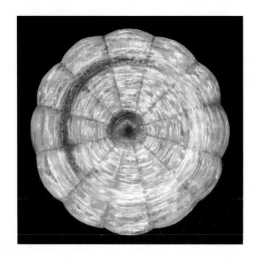

healers would claim that ill health is due to feeling separate, not a part of the whole, not in touch with the heart chakra energy. The qualities of wholeness, belonging and connection are transmitted from this centre. In addition the healer gives out an energy of love and acceptance, and all this is a powerful healing force which stimulates the heart chakra energy of the recipient. The heart chakra is governed by the thymus gland in the body, and this gland is an important part of our immune system. Strengthening the heart chakra energy also strengthens the immune system in the body.

The Fifth Chakra (Throat)

Communication is the keyword for this chakra. If you experience telepathy, verbal messages transmitted with or without an inner voice, then this chakra is functioning psychically. When the telephone rings and you know who it is before you answer, this is telepathy, as it is when you know what another person is thinking or experiencing, even though they might be far away. If you 'hear voices' that are not of the visible world, or get sounds or verbal information from a non-visible source, such as when a string of words comes into your mind seemingly from nowhere, then this is called clair-audience, which means 'clear hearing'.

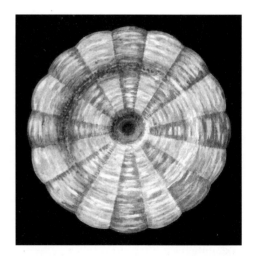

The Sixth Chakra (Eye)

Clairvoyance is the skill associated with this chakra. It means clear seeing, and it is seeing with the third eye. Any psychic information that is received visually comes through this centre, including auras and chakras. Some clairvoyants 'see' with their eyes open and some with their eyes closed. What they 'see' is an image on the third eye, which if the clairvoyant has her eyes open, will then be transposed onto the field of vision of the physical eyes. It is as though two worlds have been placed

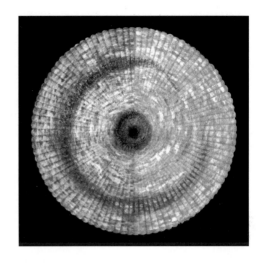

one on top of the other. The clairvoyant information doesn't exist in our physical reality, just as chakras and auras don't exist in our physical reality. They are of another realm.

The Seventh Chakra (Crown)

The crown chakra is the chakra of 'knowing', which is neither verbal nor visual. It is the chakra which understands the whole pattern, with a deep knowing understanding. It can be said to be direct inspirational knowledge from a divine source, or a clear channel into the cosmic consciousness of the universe. We probably all have experienced times when we've known exactly what to do, we've seen beyond the surface appearances to the deep underlying truth. These moments occur when we allow the crown chakra to guide us, and that potential is there all the time if we don't interfere with it.

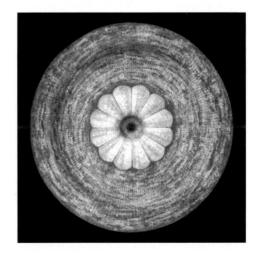

Direct control trance mediums work from this centre. These are psychics who leave their physical body and allow another being from an astral plane to enter their body and use it for a time. Books such as the 'Seth' books have been written by psychics who work in this way.

The Hand Chakras

The hands have several psychic functions. Healing comes through the hands, in conjunction with the energy of the heart chakra. The hands can heal by working on the aura of a person, or by contacting the physical body. Inspirational writing, (when a person goes into a mild trance and the writing 'takes over'), operates through the hands, in combination with the throat chakra. Psychometry, getting information by touching an object, uses the hand chakras in combination with the second, and possibly the fifth and sixth chakras. Telekinesis, the phenomenon of objects moving seemingly by themselves, can use the hand chakras in conjunction with the third chakra.

The hands are the means whereby we give out energy, and the energy we give out depends on the quality of energy flowing through the chakras. Alexander Teachers work with their hands, and the stimulus they give is related to the energy they organize through inhibition and direction of the body, and it is also related to the energy flow through the chakras. Every teacher gives a different stimulus, because we are all very different and we are giving of ourselves.

The Feet Chakras

The feet no longer have a psychic function, other than to draw the energy into the body, which is the same as their mundane function. In the bible when we hear of someone kissing another's feet, this is an indication of the healing power of the feet, which was used more in earlier times.

The Back of the Neck

The back of the neck is a very important part of our psychic mechanism. It is not a chakra as such. It is the other side of the third eye. Whereas the third eye is renowned for seeing into the future, the back of the neck can access information about the past.

It can remember our racial history and our personal past. It contacts the instinctual part of the brain, and can bring it into consciousness.

The neck is also very important in Alexander work. Freeing the neck allows a freeing to occur throughout the body. There are seven neck vertebrae, and each one of these corresponds to one of the seven chakras, so as we free the neck, we are directly stimulating a freer flow of energy through the chakras.

Psychic Alexander Teaching

During my training I was fortunate to have one teacher who often worked on the aura, and who was interested in all the subjects I am dealing with in this book. I would have

Fig. 15.1

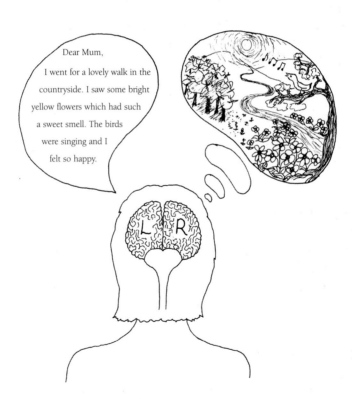

The Left and Right Hemispheres of the Brain

lessons with this teacher regularly, often going to her home to have them. When she worked aurically she was very active, waving her arms, and moving her body, almost as though she was dancing around me. One day when we had been discussing how important the 'thinking' part of the work is, and how thought doesn't exist in space-time in the same way that bodies do, we decided to try an experiment. For four or five weeks I had a 'lesson' with this teacher, but we didn't meet. I stayed at home, and lay down in semi-supine for three quarters of an hour, and noticed any sensations, feelings and changes in my body. Later when we met we would discuss what she felt she had been working on, and what I had noticed changing in my body. Our feedback always seemed to correlate. If I had noticed big changes in my legs, that would have been the area she was working on, or if it seemed to be my throat area then she too would have been thinking about, and 'dancing' around that.

I was finally convinced about this when on one occasion I lay down for my lesson in absentia and suddenly got this strong urge to get up and dance. I just didn't want to be passive, it felt wrong. So I got up and let my arms, legs, my whole body move around however it wanted to for the next three quarters of an hour. When I told her what I had done she laughed and told me she had started to work and thought, 'No, today I'm going to lie down in semi-supine'. So we had unwittingly reversed roles.

Psychism and the Left and Right Brains

There is a lot of research nowadays into the functions of the two hemispheres of our brain, and how they interact. The right brain controls the left side of the body, and the left brain the right, so for good co-ordination these two brains have to work together. The way they do work together is very complex. The left brain controls our normal everyday awareness, the verbal, deductive, rational side of our of mental skills, while the right brain controls the more visual, musical, artistic and intuitive side of us. The left brain thinks in a logical, numerical, linear way, while the right brain sees whole patterns, systems. It perceives through feelings and sensations, where the left brain works through reasoning. It synthesizes information where the left brain analyses it. Developing a kinaesthetic sense, and an awareness of the emotions and sensations in the body involves working with the right brain.

Scientific research and recent educational theory suggest that when these two hemispheres work in harmony, learning capacity and creativity are improved. What we consider 'normal' consciousness is our left-brain awareness. When a person is operating from their right brain they are often said to be in an 'altered state', or a trance state, which simply means something different from a left-brain consciousness. When we talk about the subconscious we are often talking about the activity of our right brains.

Alexander was very concerned that we learn to develop conscious control of our selves, and in this he was, albeit unwittingly, placing a great emphasis on the left brain. He deplored techniques which involved loss of conscious control, such as hypnotism. Many healing techniques use visualization and mild trance states to induce self-hypnosis and these methods were abhorrent to Alexander. These are all right-brain activities, but theories about the importance of developing the skills of the right brain were not developed in his lifetime. Nevertheless his technique did involve a process of balancing the two hemispheres of the brain. One of the aims of his work was to re-educate the use of a pupil in order that the sensory awareness of that pupil would once more become reliable. He considered the sensory awareness of a person the key to that person's vitality and wellbeing. Our kinaesthetic experiences are processed through the right brain. In effect, what Alexander taught his pupils was the development of an expanded awareness, in which the two hemispheres of the brain worked in harmony with each other. The Alexander technique encourages a constant awareness of the kinaesthetic information of the body, which is a right brain skill, while at the same time operating from choice and reason, using inhibition and direction, which are attributes of the left brain. However this expanded awareness is limited, as only some aspects of right-brain activity were acceptable to Alexander.

To be a good psychic you have to be able to use both brains together, the right brain to receive the information, intuitively, and the left brain to interpret it and communicate it verbally. It is precisely in this way that great geniuses like Einstein describe their method of thinking. In his own words:

(A) *The words or the language, as they are written or spoken, do not seem to play any role in my mechanism of thought. The psychical entities which seem to serve as elements in thought are certain signs and more or less clear images which can be 'voluntarily' reproduced and combined . . .*

(B) *The above mentioned elements are, in my case, of a visual and some of a muscular type. Conventional words or other signs have to be sought for laboriously only in a secondary stage, when the mentioned associative play is sufficiently established and can be produced at will.*

As we understand the different ways in which our minds work it will become much easier to accept the concept of psychism. Working with the left and right hemispheres

CHART SHOWING SOME OF

CHAKRAS	MUNDANE LEVEL	PHYCHIC LEVEL	COLOUR	SOUND
ROOT	Survival Instinct	Grounding Kundalini	Red	Lam
SACRAL	Emotions Pleasure Nourishment	Clairsentience	Orange	Vam
SOLAR PLEXUS	Power Achievement Success	Energy pump	Yellow	Ram
HEART	Love Acceptance Wholism	Affinity Healing	Green	Yam
THROAT	Communication Creativity	Clairaudience	Blue	Ham
EYE	Analysis World View Visualization	Clairvoyance	Indigo	Ah
CROWN	Wholism Autonomy Divinity	Knowingness	Violet	Om

of the brain is a way of balancing our intellect with our intuition. Most of us have experienced occasions when we get an intuition or a hunch, and if we act on it, it often turns out to be right. Unfortunately it's not always easy to do this because we live in a world so dominated by the scientific mode of understanding, we don't trust our intu-

THE ATTRIBUTES OF MAJOR CHAKRAS

CHAKRAS	AGE	GLANDS*	ELEMENTS	L/R BRAIN
ROOT	Infant	Gonads (Adrenals)	Earth	—
SACRAL	Child	Pancreas (Gonads)	Water	R
SOLAR PLEXUS	Adolescent	Adrenals (Pancreas)	Fire	L
HEART	Maturity	Thymus	Air	R
THROAT	Maturity	Thyroid	Ether	L + (R)
EYE	Old Age	Pituitary	Astral	L + (R)
CROWN	Death/Eternity	Pineal	Spirit	—

*There are several ways of correlating chakras with endocrine glands. I have shown alternatives.

itions. This is a cultural bias that dominates our age and society. In early Australian aboriginal society intuition was treated with extreme respect. If an Aboriginal travelling away from his family got an intuition that he should return home because something was happening at home that required his presence, then home he would go. It was as serious as getting a telegram would be for us. An Aboriginal could distinguish between intuition and 'worrying' or 'daydreaming' in a way that most of us Westerners can't. And if his intuition was seemingly 'wrong', it was never considered 'wrong', just as when a scientific experiment fails to give the required result there is always a very good reason for it. And so the cultural bias is very different.

There is a correlation between the chakras and the left and right brains. The first chakra functions by means of the autonomic nervous system. This is the part of our nervous system that functions automatically without reference to the hemispheres of the brain. Because it is an instinctual, animal part of us it does not involve conscious awareness although we can become aware of its operation when we reflect upon it. The second and fourth chakras relate to the activity of the right brain, while the third chakra relates to the left brain.

The fifth chakra is predominantly left-brained, but works with the right brain when listening to music or working psychically. The sixth chakra is also left-brained when it is thinking analytically, but rightbrained when it is visualizing or operating psychically. The crown chakra, although it includes a left and right brain function, is operating beyond the conscious brain, just as the base chakra is operating before the conscious brain.

'Seeing' The Alexander Technique

When I was training to teach the Alexander Technique we frequently had visitors to the school. They came from many different walks of life. On one occasion a man who taught psychic development visited us and he commented on what was happening at an energy level in the teaching situation. He didn't know much about the Alexander Technique, so his observations on the several teachers and students working at the school were fresh and interesting.

Firstly, he noticed that when a teacher put her hands on a student she was grounding the student by ensuring that the energy was flowing into that person from the earth. Then she was clearing and balancing the three lower chakras, in order that the energy could flow up the spine more freely. The way the teacher encouraged this upward flow was by sending messages to the student's nervous system through her hands. In this way the teacher bypassed the conscious brain, so that it could not interfere with the changes which were occurring. The lower three chakras in all the teachers were strong and well energized, and it was from these chakras that they transmitted the energizing stimulus to the students. Some teachers were also operating from the heart centre and so love and healing were coming through their hands in addition to the energy flows I have mentioned. Some of the teachers were also psychically open, and they were picking up negative energy which could be a drain upon their system because they did not know how to protect themselves.

Another visitor to the school was a Tibetan Lama, a person of advanced spiritual development. His comments were brief but to the point. What he saw happening in the school was a form of high Tantra. Tantra is a spiritual discipline in which the chakras are cleansed, purified and strengthened.

These comments and my own experience and that of many of my students suggest that the chakras are cleansed and strengthened through Alexander work. Freeing the neck and allowing the head to move forwards and up in such a way that the back lengthens and widens creates conditions in the body for a freer movement of energy up the spine and through the chakras. The energy is encouraged to move upwards, and this flow further energizes the upper chakras, and the blocks in the lower chakras begin to disperse. The direction to widen across the upper part of the arm releases the throat and heart chakras; while sending the knees forwards and away helps to ground a person and energize the root, sacral and solar plexus chakras. Even though the chakras are not physical entities themselves, they do relate to different parts of the body, and are affected by physical changes in the body and musculature. They are also affected by changes in our physical use, by developing our awareness, and by the way in which we think.

By becoming aware of habitual misuses and replacing them with improved physical use, the root chakra is cleansed, and our connection to the earth, to our roots, to the past, is brought into balance. This allows a powerful flow of earth energy to move through us, unrestricted by bad physical habits.

Refining our sensory awareness balances the second chakra. Understanding that our sensory information may be inaccurate, and needs to be balanced by our thoughts, allows cleansing and healing to take place. This lets us be in touch with our feeling awareness, and so remain centred in the present. Our feelings connect us into the present and our thoughts can lead us into the future. Wherever we put our attention, that is what we energize.

With our thoughts we can scan the possibilities of different ways of being. We can look at our options and choose. We can create a different energy flow through ourselves by giving positive attention to the option of our choice. Balancing our thoughts and our feelings refines our sensory awareness, and balances the second and third chakras.

Working with inhibition and direction develops a more positive third chakra, a powerful individual who is competent at achieving the ends she wants to gain, because of her respect for the means, the process of changing.

The principles of acceptance, non-interference and trust in the mental directions begin to develop the energy of the heart chakra.

As the lower chakras become cleansed and balanced the flow through the upper chakras becomes less distorted by interferences in the lower chakras and further growth and transformation of the self can take place.

As the lower chakras become less dominant in a person's life, and the upper chakras operate more fully, students feel the love energy of the heart centre altering their emotional attitude to life; often students feel the need to be more creative because the throat chakra is more stimulated. As the energy stimulates the brow and crown chakras, the student finds her perspective on life is changing, and often a spiritual searching begins.

The Alexander Technique is a way of learning to use your mind and body well. It is a way of bringing the whole person into balance. Many people come to the Alexander Technique because they have some specific problem that they want to 'sort out', an end that they want to gain, such as a bad back, a tension problem and so on. But many are attracted to the Alexander Technique because they realize it is doing much more than sorting out a particular problem. Usually, as a result of a few lessons, a student notices changes in herself which she is unable to put into words. She may say she feels more balanced, calmer, less easily thrown. The changes that are happening are much deeper than most students anticipate, and these non-specific changes in the 'being nature' of a person are one of the most important reasons why many students continue with the Alexander Technique, and why more and more people decide to train to be teachers. They notice changes of a fundamental kind taking place. These changes are difficult to put into words because they are about an aspect of life we don't often talk or even think about. In a sense they are not about an aspect of life at all, but about the source of it.

Looking at the way you use yourself, and working at releasing any blocks that interfere with good use, can cause changes to take place in a person at a very deep and fundamental level. Of course it is always up to the individual to choose how deeply she wants to work with this technique, and for some people the Alexander Technique is a simple and effective method of keeping the mind and body functioning well, through inhibition and giving the appropriate directions in all situations. For others the work opens up emotional, psychological and spiritual questions that need to be dealt with in their own right.

Chapter Sixteen

Looking After Your Energy System

As we become aware of ourselves as much much more than a physical body, then we need to learn ways of taking care of that larger whole. Just as we feed, clean, exercise and rest our bodies, we need an equivalent for our thoughts, feelings, and all the other energic parts of our being. We need the energy system to function as well as it can. Einstein's theory of relativity has led to an understanding of the world no longer in terms of 'things', but in terms of 'relationships'. In the same way when we talk about ourselves as an energy system, that energy system is an aspect of a larger energy system, which is the earth, and in turn the earth is a part of the energy system of the universe.

Within our system we are constantly influenced by our own different energies, as our bodies, thoughts and feelings change, and in addition we are constantly interacting with energies around us. I have found that using the theory of the chakras is a most helpful way of understanding how to bring the different energies into balance.

Ian rang me up one day to ask me if I could help him. He had had his arm amputated above the elbow as a result of a motorbike accident, and suffered from constant phantom pain in the missing arm. He was twenty years old. I said I really didn't know if I would be able to help him, but if he wanted to give it a try then he was welcome to come along and see me. So he did.

The only time Ian wasn't in pain was when he was asleep, and for the first ten minutes on waking in the morning. The pain in the missing arm and hand came in cycles, each cycle lasting two or three minutes, building from mild pain to extreme pain, in the missing hand and lower arm.

Ian needed a lot of Alexander work. Not only was his left arm amputated, which meant that his right shoulder carried most of the weight of the artificial arm, but his left leg had been damaged in the accident and had not regained its strength. The right side of Ian's body was doing all the work, so he was very out of balance, with a tendency to over-contracted musculature on the right and energic disconnection in the left leg.

When I worked near the amputated arm I felt a strong energy field around it, so I began working on this. When I worked on his aura around the missing arm I could either increase the level of pain or diminish it, and when I diminished it, Ian would move into a very relaxed trance state, sometimes falling asleep. It became clear that the pain decreased when I worked to release or neutralize the energy from the energy field around the missing arm. I could feel exactly where in the missing arm I was working to release the energy, and so could Ian. It seemed that because Ian no longer had a hand, the energy could not release out of the hand chakra normally, and the build up of energy caused the pain. But if I gently pulled the energy through the 'missing arm and hand' and out of the system then the pain would diminish and for periods of about twenty minutes it would go away altogether.

This hypothesis seemed to be backed up by the fact that the arm hurt least when Ian was least energized, asleep or just awakened, and the pain was worst when Ian was active, playing squash for instance. The medical explanation for Ian's pain was that the nerves were badly damaged when the arm was ripped off by a lorry. If I worked on the muscles around the wound the intensity of the pain became extreme, because I was stimulating the damaged nerves, and energizing the arm, whereas if I worked on the energy field and released energy from the arm I could quieten the nerves, reduce the pain, and for a short time stop it altogether. So I restricted my hands-on work to the rest of his body and worked aurically on the damaged arm.

I showed Ian what I was doing aurically around his amputated arm, so that he could do it too, and he found he could reduce the intensity of the pain by working on himself in this way. He also learnt how to ground himself, especially through the left leg, and this also helped to release the build up of excess energy. He never completely cured the pain, but he learned how to control the level of it, so that it was not as extreme.

Active and Passive Energy States

When we are active, no matter through which chakra, working, singing, dancing, expressing emotion, thinking purposefully, then our energy is radiating out. The aura is energized by the activity of the chakras. When our energy is radiating outwards, less energy can enter into the aura because it is full of our own energy. On the other hand when we are passive, daydreaming, watching television, reading, getting in touch with what is going on inside us, then we are more open to outside influences. Our energy is not radiating out, so other vibrations enter the aura.

Some psychically sensitive people pick up energies around them, and this tendency can develop when a person begins studying the Alexander Technique. Firstly, when people begin working with the technique, they start directing their attention inwards upon themselves, probably much more than usual, as they refine their self awareness. They are operating in a receptive 'listening' state more often, inhibiting habitual responses, learning to 'do' less and 'allow' more. This makes them much more open to influences entering their aura.

Secondly the interferences in the chakras are being slowly dissolved away by the work with the Alexander Technique, and this means that there is more energy flowing in the system, which may increase the psychic functioning of some people. Also, as the energy flow changes in the chakras, problems which previously were 'buried' become energized, brought into consciousness, and have to be dealt with.

Interferences Attract Energy

The energic interferences in the chakra system can operate rather like electro-magnets. They attract energy from outside into the system, which will help the chakra to be stimulated, and the blockage to be dissolved. We respond to an interference either by being attracted or repelled. Attraction can be felt as love, or excitement. Repulsion can be experienced as hatred or fear or hostility. All these attitudes attract outside 'attention' or energy.

For example if a person has a block in the second chakra about sexuality, he will tend either to be obsessive about sex or to avoid sex totally. The chakra will be overactive or underactive. If the person is avoiding the problem, this may work while the person operates predominantly in the active mode, but it is impossible to be continuously active, and if in addition he begins developing his receptivity through Alexander lessons, then he may attract energy into his aura that will stimulate that chakra. He will experience this as being attracted to people who help him in one way or another (pleasant or unpleasant), to face the problem. The root of the problem will be to do with his inability to experience deep contact and nourishment. Until he has learnt how to experience fulfilment in terms of nourishment and pleasure the interference will continue to attract energy into it. If he is not aware why this is happening he may keep repeating past mistakes by reacting habitually to the stimulus.

Alternatively if a person feels he is a victim, there is interference to the flow of energy in the third chakra, and he will attract 'victim' situations to him, energy that could be used to learn the lessons of the third chakra and disperse the blockage if he is aware of what is going on.

Our aura could be like a protective energy field. It is possible to experience the energy, positive or negative, entering the aura and allow it to flow through the aura and pass out again. This attitude of non-resistance simply allows the energy to flow undisturbed. But if there are blocks in the chakras they suck the appropriate energy into them, through attraction or repulsion, in order to heal the blockage. If there were no interferences it would be possible to go into a room and feel the vibrations at an auric level, and consciously choose whether we wish to open psychically to those vibrations or not. Some rooms feel wonderful and it is good to open the chakras and receive the energy into them. We often do this automatically. When we experience a gentle sigh, it is often a sign that the heart chakra has opened a little, because some loving heart energy has entered the aura.

Some of the exercises in this section can be used to help protect yourself from unwanted outside influences. But it is important to be aware that when we pick up negative energies it is something from within our own energy systems that attracts them. It is pointless to blame the other energies out there for polluting us. If all our chakras were flowing freely, without interference, it would simply be a matter of conscious choice whether we stayed with an energy or let go of it. Our fears and our needs pull the energy into the chakras, whether we like it or not.

There can be a danger of being obsessive about self-protection too. Many of the exercises on psychic protection effectively cut a person off from all outside influences, and ultimately that means cutting off from relationship altogether, not a desirable end for anyone.

However most of us have lots of problems, lots of interferences to an easy flow of the energy through us, and it helps to be able to look after our system as it is now, to know how to feed and nourish it, how to cleanse it, how to exercise and rest it, and how to protect it whenever we feel that is necessary.

The Effect of Alexander Work

If you find you are one of the people who becomes more psychically open as a result of Alexander work it may be especially important to work with the following exercises. Working with the Alexander Technique you are learning to balance your energies in many different ways. Your Alexander Teacher will be helping you to release muscle imprinting, to let go of old muscular habits which were part of your defences. All this will be affecting the energy in the chakras and encouraging the interferences to dissolve away. For a time you may feel very vulnerable, as though you are semi-permeable, with no defences. If this is your experience, then it can be a very worrying part of the process of changing. It may be helpful to get reassurance from other people who have been through this stage, that it does not last forever, and that it is worth the difficulties.

As you refine your self-awareness, your energy system becomes more sensitive and, for a time, more easily thrown out of balance. You need to be able to balance your inward and outward energy, to give and to receive, and yet to choose whether or not to receive certain energies that may be painful and unpleasant for you, and how to cleanse yourself and let the negative energies inside you release and disperse. You may feel you need to take responsibility for the energy you radiate outwards to the world. At this time it is most important to know how to cleanse, strengthen and protect your energy system, and you would benefit a great deal if you developed a daily practice of 'psychic hygiene'.

All the following exercises are ones that I have found helpful in my work. Firstly it is important to pause, and become aware of what is happening. Get to know what your energy habits are. Are you too open, or too closed, or ungrounded, or something else? When you feel you understand your habits you are in a better position to give mental directions to alter your energy state, letting go of what is no longer helpful and introducing a new means whereby you can operate energically.

CLEANSING EXERCISES

There are lots of cleansing exercises. I shall mention one or two, but I recommend that you make up your own. You can swim in golden pools, walk through cleansing mists, anything you like, as long as it has a 'good cleansing feeling' about it.

Physical washing is always a good way of cleansing the whole energy system. Water is a cleansing element, so showering or bathing is very good. Even washing your hands can change the energy in your system.

• *Aura Cleansing* •

If you feel you've just walked into some difficult energy, anywhere, this can be a useful way of clearing it.

Imagine you are a chicken, with feathers, and that what you have picked up has ruffled your feathers. Brush them down again, all over your body, partly touching yourself and partly not. You may notice areas where the energy doesn't feel smooth, and you have to stroke the feathers down there, more than anywhere else. Trust these intuitions. Finally be sure to brush under the bottom of your feet (or shoes), as this clears your contact with the earth.

• *The Energy Shower* •

A useful habit to develop is to imagine that at any time you wish you can switch on a tap, and receive a shower of golden rain to cleanse you. I recommend installing one of these showers above your front door, so while you search for your key, you can switch on the energy shower above the door, and clean yourself down before you enter the house, leaving any bad vibrations you picked up outside, soaking back down into the earth. (*Fig. 16.1*)

• *Chakra Cleansing* •

If it is warm and dry enough for you to do this visualization exercise outdoors, so you really are in contact with the earth below you, then I recommend you do so. However, it is also effective indoors.

Lie down in the prone position. If you find this position uncomfortable it may help to have a cushion under your chest and tummy. Feel the contact of your body against the earth. Lie quietly listening to your breathing. Allow yourself to relax into the ground. Go through some of your bodyscanning exercises until you are feeling more in touch with your body.

Bring your attention to the coccyx at the base of the spine. Visualize the base chakra concealed in this part of you. Imagine that as you give attention to it you can see a door, and you know if you open the door you will get a picture or a symbol of your base chakra. Open the door and note what you see. The image you get may be a positive or negative one. It may give you some insight into yourself, at a base chakra level - how you relate to your survival instincts, and your raw energy supply. Now imagine that coming out of the sky down into your hand is a hosepipe, and out of it pours beautiful golden water. This water is cosmic cleansing energy, and you can use it to clean out the base chakra. If the image of the base chakra was healthy and positive, then this golden water will nourish and energize it even more. Even if you had an image of a fire, this golden water will not put it out. It will cleanse it and leave it burning all the more brightly. If your image was more negative, then let the golden water wash it clean away, washing out any dirty corners of the chakra, any blocks and interferences, until the negative image is replaced by a vortex of glowing red light.

Move to the second chakra and repeat this process, opening a door at the sacral area of the spine, finding a symbol or image to give you insight into this chakra, and then cleansing the chakra with golden liquid, until it is glowing orange, and the image is either enhanced or washed away.

Repeat this process through all the chakras, using the colours of the rainbow as they correspond to each chakra (see chart pages 230-231).

When you have cleansed all the chakras and let all the rubbish in them fall down into the earth, give your attention to your body and your aura. Direct the golden water into the air, so it comes down in a beautiful shower all over your body, and all around it. Let this golden rain carry away any dirt, any dis-ease, anything you would like to be cleansed away. Let it pour down into the earth, until your whole body is shining with golden light, and with the coloured lights of the chakras shining up and down the spine and head of the body.

Now stand up and move around a little, and then find a different spot to lie down on. Once again lie down in

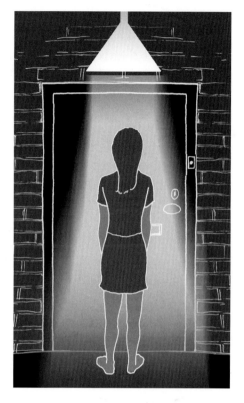

Fig. 16.1 The Energy Shower

prone, and this time soak up the earth energy into your body. Imagine the earth energy as white light, and feel its strong healthy energy filling your base chakra, then your sacral chakra, then your solar plexus chakra, and so on until all the chakras are filled with both golden (cosmic) and earth (white) light. Let the white light fill your body, and radiate out into your aura. Really experience your connection with the life-sustaining earth, as you become aware of its energy filling you.

When you are ready, stand up and continue feeling the white light flowing up through your feet, legs, trunk, down your arms and out of your hands, and through your neck and out of the top of your head. Visualize the golden light flowing down through your head, neck and trunk, down your arms and out through your hands, and down your legs and out through your feet. Let the light flow into your body and into your aura.

Think of your neck being free, and the head moving forwards and up. Imagine that the energy flowing through your system is allowing this to happen, as it allows the back to lengthen and widen, and the shoulder and pelvic girdles to release. Continue to give your directions, experiencing yourself as an energy system, energized by your own thought and attention. Visualize the chakras glowing their different colours right up the length of your body, allowing lengthening and widening as they open and expand.

You can vary this exercise according to personal taste. Some people prefer not to lie in prone, and it can be done in sitting, standing, or lying in semi-supine. I find the experience of releasing the chakras into the earth is particularly powerful in prone, as is receiving the earth energy into the chakras in this position. You may not find it necessary to change position, when you change from releasing into the earth, to receiving from it, but a lot of people get very confused because they start imagining they are bringing all their rubbish back into the system, and so moving to different part of the earth removes that unhelpful thought process.

• Space Cleansing •

There are lots of rituals for cleansing a room or some other space. Burning incense, a candle, or the herb sage, is effective. These rituals come from ancient religious traditions, both Western and North American Indian.

Alternatively you can visualize white light filling the room, starting from the earth below and streaming out of the windows and ceiling. Or you may work out a good visualization of your own.

GROUNDING AND CENTERING

At a physical level we are all part of the earth. That physical part comes from the earth and returns to it when we die. When we have a good relationship with the earth we know our fundamental survival needs will be met. We experience our world as a supportive place. We comfortably allow the ground to take our weight, and in response the earth energy flows easily into our feet and root chakras and from there throughout the body. When this is happening we are well grounded.

Centering is very similar to grounding. Centering is focused on the second chakra, whereas grounding is focused on the first, and the two are very connected. The Centre of Gravity of the body as a whole is at the same position as the second or sacral chakra. This chakra is also called the Hara and in Martial Arts it is the point out of which any movement of the body takes place. It is the fulcrum or the point of balance of the body. And so our weight which connects us downwards into the earth, through the root and feet chakras, is centred in the sacral chakra. The two chakras affect each other a great deal because if a person is ungrounded they will also be uncentred, and if a person is uncentred they often become ungrounded.

When we are centred we are content simply living in the here and now. This moment in time, this place, these people, being in this body, doing this activity or doing nothing, all feel very satisfying. If we are grounded we are confident that our physical needs are being met. If we are centred we are confident that our emotional needs are being met. When we are well centred in the sacral chakra we are strongly in touch with our feelings,

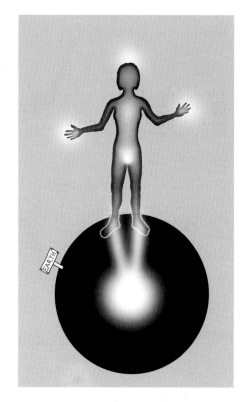

Fig. 16.2 Grounding and Centering

emotional and physical, and thus able to use them as a reference point for the rest of our activities, physical, emotional, mental and spiritual, that is, for the energies of the higher chakras. If the second chakra is in a good state, then all our activities come from an essential sense of wellbeing, of trust in the 'rightness' of things, of confidence that life is a satisfying and nourishing experience.

Recipe for being Centred

Enjoy who you are,
Enjoy who you are with,
Enjoy where you are,
Enjoy what you do.

Fig. 16.3

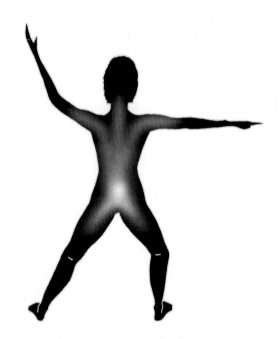

Martial Arts energize the sacral chakra

Our energy system as a whole is much more than a body, and there are times when it doesn't make a good connection with the earth, usually times when life is more difficult physically or emotionally, and part of us literally doesn't want to be here. Then the subtle body begins to split away from the physical body at the root and sacral chakras. We often become ungrounded because we are uncentred, the emotional problems creating the stress and fear that makes the subtle body split away.

When a person is ungrounded she often tightens in the legs, and in the powerful muscles that connect the front of the legs into the spine.

When these muscles release they often cause a release in the muscle of the diaphragm. Often, a sign of returning to groundedness is a deep releasing breath, that feels like a great relief!

Jane had sciatica for five years. When I worked on her I found her legs energically disconnected, so she was very ungrounded. She responded well to energy work and I worked on her aura for most of the session. I gave her lots of grounding exercises. She got rid of her sciatica overnight, and during the next two years she had lessons with me it never returned, and as far as I know it hasn't done since she stopped having lessons. She simply needed the tools with which to work on her own ungroundedness.

Not all sufferers of sciatica are ungrounded. There are lots of other reasons for sciatica, and lower back pain in general, but this is an important one, which I have come across several times.

If the second chakra is disturbed, which tends to be one of the patterns of our culture, then our behaviour has not got a self-satisfied reference point. We act from needs and bitterness, sadness and longings. Our attention would rather be anywhere than in touch with that feeling reality. We want to become this person who looks so happy and glamourous, or we want to be six months further on from today when everything is going to be alright, or we want to be in Australia, anywhere, rather than 'Me, Here, Now'.

For many of us, the process of becoming centred takes time, working on the emotions in the way I have described in earlier chapters, and letting go of old pains and traumas that distort the energy through this centre. The following exercises help to shift attention to the second chakra. As you energize it you may become aware of some of the interferences to its easy flow.

When a person is ungrounded and uncentred she tends to live in her thoughts rather than her feelings. She may be preoccupied with the past, nostalgically or bitterly, or by the future, excitedly or fearfully. Thoughts of one sort or another block out the sensations and emotions of the present. She feels 'spaced out', out of touch with reality, living in a fantasy world. All these are symptoms of being ungrounded. For some people being ungrounded is such an habitual experience that it seems normal. This is an example of their faulty sensory appreciation.

The following exercises should be experimented with to find which type of exercise suits you, and gives you a stronger feeling of connection with the earth energy and with your centre.

• 1. Let The Earth Ground You •

It usually grounds people if they get out into the countryside, and one of the best ways of grounding yourself is to hug a tree. Find a tree that looks strong and healthy and let the whole front (or back) part of your body rest against the tree, and feel the energy of this most grounded of living beings. Incidentally this just won't work if you feel self-conscious, because that very embarrassment will be encouraging you to leap out of your body again, and not 'be here', which is ungrounding, so if you're the shy type, be sure to find a spot where you feel safe, either amongst understanding friends, or unobserved. (*Fig. 16.4*)

Fig. 16.4

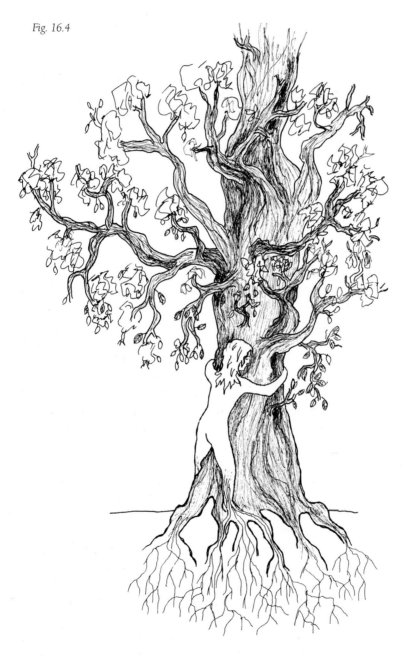

Hugging a Tree

• 2. Enjoy Your Feet and Legs •

Another simple way of grounding yourself is to go through the exercise on pages 38-39, in which you stroke, massage and pat each foot and ankle, calf and knee, thigh and hip, in turn. Giving all this physical, emotional and mental attention to your legs can be a very effective grounding method.

• 3. Tree Visualization •

See the grounding exercise on page 206

• 4. Sending Down a Grounding Cord •

I find this a useful exercise to do at any time when I am feeling ungrounded. You can do it sitting in a meeting, in a car or a bus, standing in a queue, at any time when you feel it might help you.

Imagine that there is a tube, like a fireman's hose, which you can see hanging down from the base of your spine, going down, down into the earth, until it is about a half a mile inside the earth. This is your grounding cord. If it helps you can place an anchor on the end of this cord, to encourage it to go down into the earth. This is your connection into the earth energy. Up the outside of the tube travels the earth energy, into your feet, legs and base chakra. Down the centre of the tube you can send any energy in your body that you don't want there, any pain, any anxiety, any anger or disturbance of any kind. If you feel you've picked up negative energy from outside, then send it down the tube. Imagine the tube to be rather like the rabbit hole that Alice dropped down. See little clusters of unwanted energy floating easily down that hole to return to the earth. If they won't float down, hang weights on to them to pull them down into the earth.

The better able you are to visualize this tube descending into the ground (even if it has to go through several floors of a building first - just picture it doing that), the better grounded you will be. If the visualization has a feeling quality to it, as though you really do believe it is there because you can feel it, then it will be all the more effective.

When you have sent the grounding cord down, you may notice a change in your state as your body contacts the earth energy more strongly. You may find you are suddenly breathing more deeply. If you now add the Alexander directions to the grounding directions, you may find an even better change of state developing, as your body responds appreciatively to the positive mental directions you are giving it.

• 5. 'Seeing' Your Feet and Legs •

Lie down in semi-supine, and when you are feeling calm and rested, give your attention to each leg in turn. Notice how the left foot is resting against the floor. How does the knee joint feel? How does the hip joint feel? How do the fleshy parts of the leg feel? How does the leg connect into the trunk of the body? Does it feel as though it really belongs to you or not? Now visualize the energy flowing from the earth into the foot, the leg and the pelvis, energizing the base chakra, and then flowing up the spine and out of the head. Does the energy flow easily through the leg? Can you feel or see points where there are interferences to an easy flow? Now go through the same process with the right leg. Notice the differences between the two legs.

This exercise may give you insights into how you habitually ground yourself. Perhaps one leg may seem much more strongly connected to the earth than the other. Remember that this work is imaginative, and your sensory appreciation may not be accurate. Nevertheless it is a valuable way of getting to know how you feel about your legs and your grounding. If you are working with a teacher, tell her what your feelings and images were and she may be able to clarify the picture for you with her feedback.

After getting the visual picture of each leg, work with the visualization in order to get the energy flowing strongly through both legs, into the base chakra, up the spine, and out of the head. If you felt there were blocks to the energy flow, work to change the visual picture so that the energy is moving freely through the blocked part. Cleanse the blockages using the hosepipe of golden rain that you used to clean your chakras (see page 240). Then see if the new visualization can actually be linked to a feeling of energy flowing through the legs. Linking visualization with feeling in this way is very powerful, and can bring about a lot of change.

• 6. Golden Rain •

The golden water of the shower of the chakra cleansing exercise can help with grounding, if you imagine the water flowing down though your body and filling up your legs, until your legs are full of water, and then letting the water pour out into the earth as more water flows in from the top. I find this exercise works best in standing or sitting. (*Fig. 16.5*)

• 7. Enjoy Your Self •

One of the simplest ways of grounding and centering yourself is to do something which your body likes doing. It may be swimming, or dancing, or making love. Also you may like to consult the list of all the things that give you pleasure and find something which will nourish and centre you (see page 208).

• 8. Your Head, Your Feet and Your Centre •

Stand or sit quietly, pausing and noticing how you are feeling, grounding yourself in some way, and giving your Alexander directions, so you are becoming more self-aware. Be aware of three important parts of your body.

   a. Your head, on a free neck, being in a forwards and up direction, your contact with heaven, with the upward flow.
   b. Your feet contacting the earth, your grounding contact, connecting also with your base chakra.
   c. Your 'guts', your second chakra, the centre of gravity of your body, your centre, balancing you physically and emotionally.

   Notice the difference in sensations and emotions as you move your attention from one of these parts to the next. If you can work with a partner, it is quite interesting to work with this exercise together. As one person focuses on one area the other person can give that person a push, as though to push her over, (not too hard!). Notice the difference in stability according to where your attention is focused.
   When you have focused separately on the different areas, give attention to all three at the same time, with the following thoughts.

   My head leads me forwards and upwards, into the future.
   My feet hold me backwards and downwards connecting into the past.
   My guts are where I am now, right here, in the present.

• 9. The Lake •

Sit in a supportive chair. Put your hands in a cupped shape over your second chakra area and give it all your attention. Be aware of your body moving out in all directions from this space, and your aura spreading out even further beyond your body. Feel that you are at the centre of your aura. Be aware of your breathing and visualize the breath entering your body like a mist, and then turning into a liquid, which flows right down into your second chakra. Your second chakra is a beautiful still lake, being filled more and more completely with each breath. Feel that you are cupping that beautiful still lake with your hands. Keep doing this for some time, allowing the centred feeling to become more and more intense.

• 10. Double Attention •

After getting into the centred state described in the above exercise, begin to explore the environment around you. Don't allow your attention to be totally caught up in what you are looking at, always keep part of your attention on the second chakra, where your hands are still cupped. Notice if you lose your centre at any point. Then get up from standing, and begin walking around, keeping an awareness of your whole body moving, giving your Alexander directions, and maintaining a centre of consciousness in the second chakra, while also looking at the environment around you. Go for a walk in the town, watching the world around you from that centred place, always keeping a state of double attention, watching yourself inside, and the world outside. Notice if this feels any different from your normal awareness and in what way.

• Staying Grounded and Centred with Other People Around •

The hardest test for maintaining centredness is when you are with other people. Other people are so distracting! Remember they are very powerful energy systems, which interact with your energy in all sorts of ways. You may be attracted to them, hate them, be afraid of what they may think about you and so on. The distractions to remaining in that calm self-satisfied second chakra space are endless. It is a very good exercise to practise giving your directions, staying in your centre, at the centre of your aura, in control of your space, and yet attentive to the people around you at the same time. Notice the difference in comparison to your usual behaviour.

This ability to maintain a double attention to the inside and the outside world is at the centre of the Alexander Technique, and it is also central to all psychic work.

If you find you often tend to lose your centre when you are with another person, it may be because you are a psychically open person. The chances are you have merged your aura with the other person, your attention has leapt right out of your body and into the other persons, and you are no longer in touch with who you are as a separate being. If your habit is to identify totally with the other person, then a useful exercise would be to note ten things that you do not have in common with her or him. In addition to the exercises on grounding and centering the following exercises on how to open and close the chakras, and how to protect yourself psychically, will be helpful.

• *Opening and Closing the Psychic Level of the Chakras* •

This book is not intended to teach the reader how to operate at a psychic level, so the 'Opening' exercise is not sufficient in itself to develop a psychic level of awareness in a person. It is a very powerful exercise which will energize the chakras at a mundane level, and it may open them at a psychic level. My interest is in the reader who often finds himself psychically open and wishes to close down at the psychic level. However I feel I cannot give the 'Closing' exercise without giving the 'Opening' one first, and I cannot overemphasize the importance of closing down carefully every time you do the 'Opening' exercise.

• *Opening* •

Sit comfortably on a straight backed chair. Think of your sitting bones and your feet in contact with the floor, your neck being free, and the head going forwards and up, so that the back lengthens and widens, widening across the upper part of the arms and sending the knees forwards and away. Don't let the Alexander directions be a 'fix'. After you have given them, have the sense that your body is carrying out the directions 'softly', that the muscles are released, not held or tense. Think that it is easy to give the directions and that your body is easy as it responds to them.

Once again put your attention on your sitting bones, your feet, your points of contact with the earth. Now send down your grounding cord (see pages 247-48).

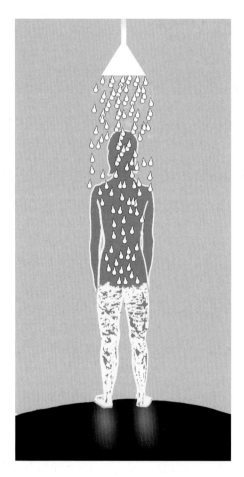

Fig. 16.5 Grounding with Golden Rain

Notice your breathing. Imagine every time you breathe you are drawing the energy down into the root chakra. The root is also being fed by energy from the feet chakras and from the grounding cord. Visualize the breath coming in through the feet and the grounding cord as well as down through the mouth and throat, and the breath, like a white light converging upon the root chakra and energizing it. At a psychic level the root chakra is always open, energizing the rest of the system. See the root chakra as a beautiful flower which glows brighter and brighter as you energize it, the white light filling the whole of the pelvic area. A lotus flower is the traditional image, but you could imagine any flower you choose. You may like to visualize a different type of flower for each chakra.

Keep breathing into the root chakra like this for several breaths. Don't force the breathing. Simply allow it to happen. Visualize your root chakra becoming more and more energized. Now, on the next breath visualize the energy entering the root chakra and then being pushed up a transparent tube in the centre of the spine until it arrives at the second chakra, where the white light energy opens out the second chakra.

See the second chakra as a flower in bud, and as the white light reaches it the bud of the flower opens out until it becomes a fully expanded flower glowing with white light, the light filling the whole of the lower abdominal area. Continue directing the breath into the root chakra, so both chakras become fully energized, and then allow the white light to travel up the transparent tube to the third chakra at the solar plexus region.

Go through the same process with the third chakra. Notice physical changes, and sensations as you open each chakra. Continue breathing into the root chakra, and being aware that each chakra that you have opened is a fully opened flower, glowing brightly.

When the flower of the third chakra is fully opened and glowing move up to the heart chakra. Notice the subtle changes that occur as you move up through the chakras. There will probably be an increasing sense of expansion at each chakra level of the body. When you open the throat chakra you may experience ringing in your ears, and when you move to the eye centre it may feel quite tight around the forehead. Finally move up to the crown chakra, which, like the base chakra is always open, and allow the white light to flow through it into the universe. At the same time see golden light pouring down into your body from above through the crown chakra, and through all the other chakras, also through your whole body and your aura. Let the golden light carry away any impurities or unwanted stuff down through the grounding cord and the feet into the centre of the earth.

You are now open and ready to work psychically, but as I have already said I do not think it is within the scope of this book to go into what to do next! It is important to be aware when you open in this way that you are making yourself open to many influences, some good and some not so good. At this point I always feel it is appropriate to give thanks and to ask for guidance from the divine source, whatever that may mean to you, and to offer whatever skills you may have for the good of humankind and the universe as a whole.

• Closing Down •

Learning how to close down the chakras is much more important than learning how to open them up. In many people they open up automatically. You just have to mention the word 'psychic' and they're off! So here's how to put them to bed.

Using the image of the open chakras with all the flowers open and glowing, you are now going to reverse the process. Do the closing down exercise quickly and always do it twice. Doing it quickly gets you out of the meditative altered state that encourages psychic opening. Doing it twice means that you haven't done it so quickly that it's not effective.

The crown chakra always remains open, feeding your whole being with cosmic energy, so begin with the eye chakra and close it down into a tight little bud with not one drop of light left around it. Watch the light going down the transparent tube to the throat chakra, so that section of the tube is now completely dark. Now close down the throat chakra in the same way, until it is a tight dark little bud, and let the energy flow down into the heart chakra, which you close down in the same way.

Carry on with this process down through the lower chakras. These are the ones that particularly like to stay open, so be sure they are well closed. You may have to put a strap round the bud, and you may even have to padlock it! Use any image that gets the light out of the system, and the flower closed into a tight bud. The root chakra like the crown chakra stays open, so you only have five chakras to deal with. Make sure they are all well closed down, and then do it again and again until you are confident there's not one drop of light left in the system.

Don't worry that by closing the psychic level of, say, the heart chakra you are also closing it at a mundane level. You're not. Your being knows what you want, so as you think the thoughts of closing down psychically that's exactly what it will do. You will probably feel a narrowing and an internal 'darkening' as you do this exercise. That's good. When you've finished, get up and move around. Feel yourself back on the earth plane.

• *Alternative image* •

If you don't like seeing the chakra as a flower, you may like to work with some other image such as a glowing source of light, or a spinning light, rather like the 'Catherine wheel' firework.

PROTECTION

All the exercises we have covered above are forms of self-protection at an energy level. In order to protect our energy systems and keep them in a good state, we need to be grounded, centred, we need to know how to cleanse psychically, and we need to know how to close down the psychic mechanism.

I have already explained why sometimes it is useful to be able to protect oneself at an energy level. If you can imagine a perfect enlightened being, like a Buddha or a Christ figure, grounded, centred, and connected through the crown chakra to the cosmic flow of energy, with no blocks in any of the chakras to interfere with that flow, then the energy passing into that being's energy system would simply flow through. It would flow through, neither attracted here nor resisted there, just accepted, received and let go of. The person would be transparent, radiating out her own beingness, the energy of her chakra system simply being what it is. This person would have no need of protection. 'Difficult' energy would flow through this radiant being and in doing so it would be transformed by the energy of her system and flow out again no longer as difficult energy.

Well, we can't all turn into perfect radiant beings overnight. We might not even want to. It may be just fine to be exactly how we are, with all our faults and imperfections, but this means we must take responsibility for what we experience at an energy level, because we are attracting that experience into our systems. However one very good way of learning to protect oneself is to work with the above model, of transparency and non-resistance to the energy flows that enter one's space.

• 1. Developing Non-Resistance and Transparency •

Imagine you are transparent. You may like to use the imagery of modern science fiction, and become 'beamed up', or you can imagine your body is a window or a pure crystal. Allow that transparent awareness to extend into your aura too, so you are visualizing yourself as a pure energy system. Whatever energy comes into your auric space, flows through it, flows through your body, and flows out the other side and away. You don't encourage it in, you don't resist it entering your energy field. You just let it pass.

It is interesting to work with this model whenever you are in a situation where there is 'difficult' energy around but it hasn't got a lot to do with you: if, for example you are in a supermarket and a row breaks out with people getting angry and upset. If that sort of situation sometimes upsets you, try becoming transparent and letting the energy flow through you. If you find that works well for you, you could then go on to try this way of being in difficult situations that are more close to home.

One of the best times to use it, if you are able, is when someone you are very close to is angry and upset with you for some reason. She may need to express her emotion. If it is possible to allow her to do that without it sparking off your emotions, by just letting her pure emotion flow through you and out and away, without resisting it, or encouraging it, then it will be very helpful to her and to the relationship. But this must be a genuine non-reaction. If you are pretending to be a perfect being it will feel very condescending and will not help you to understand your own genuine responses. But people who have learnt to work with this honestly have found it very helpful in relationships, a good way to stop molehills turning into mountains.

Non-resistance is a form of inhibition. It is the ability not to respond to a stimulus. It is the middle path of non-doing, where you neither react nor resist reacting, and it is partly because this effortless middle path is so hard to reach that many people have problems understanding 'inhibition'. It is so easy to turn it into repression, which is a form of resistance.

On those days when you don't feel up to being transparent, and dealing with difficult energies by non-resistance, then there are protective techniques which develop one's resistance to energy entering the energy field. As long as you are clear that that is what you are doing then you can choose which response is going to work best for you in any situation.

• 2. *Closing Down and Zipping Up* •

In addition to closing down the chakras, imagine that there is a zip fastener running up the length of the chakras which you can zip up, or zip down if you prefer. There is also a small zip running down the back of the neck, which you can zip up, as energy can enter in through here too. Although it is not a chakra, each vertebra of the neck corresponds to a chakra, and energy can get into the system in this way.

• 3. *Circle of Light* •

Surround yourself with a circle of white light which contains you and your aura, like a bubble. You can also place a circle of white light, with a cross inside it, in front of each chakra, as extra protection. (*Fig. 16.6*)

• 4. *Protective Clothing* •

A blue cloak, still traditionally the uniform of the nurse, is an ancient symbol of protection which you can visualize covering you. For the more modernistically inclined a space-suit is quite a powerful symbol of protection.

• 5) *Sending the Energy Away* •

If you feel you have difficult energy inside you which you can't get rid of, then there are several options.

Send the energy down your grounding cord, or back to where it came from. If you feel you are full of another person's energy, not necessarily good or bad energy, just not yours, then imagine gathering all that energy into a ball and throwing it back to the person it belongs to.

If that doesn't work, then you may need to do some work with this energy, as outlined in Chapter 11, 'The Emotional Body'.

Disembodied Beings

You may feel there is energy around you coming from some energy form that is not physical. People give lots of names to disembodied beings, and there can be good or bad ones: spirit guides, lower or higher astral beings, ghosts. I do not wish to discuss these entities in any depth. I have no doubt that some of my readers will hear voices and experience these entities around them. I think it is only a matter of time before we get more concrete evidence of their existence, as we now have evidence of auras and chakras. However I do recommend that if you do hear voices, or receive 'guidance', you do not listen uncritically, but with the discrimination and wisdom with which you would listen to guidance from a living physical being. If the guidance feels right to you, then act upon it, and take responsibility for your action, but if it feels wrong, then don't act upon it. If you treat a disembodied being as though it were a god (guide), then you may have some third chakra stuff to deal with, for you are giving away your power, and potentially becoming a victim. Treat an entity as you would treat a person you want an equal relationship with. In time you may decide the entity is very wise, or you may decide it is very foolish. Such judgements take time. If you invest it with more power than you, you are acting out the victim.

If you feel the entity is very unwise, or if you feel there is energy coming from an entity which is very difficult, as is the case with some ghosts, then send the entity away. Tell it in an authoritative voice to go back to where it belongs. If it doesn't work, you may need to find professional help from an experienced person. A professional clairvoyant or your local spiritualist church may know of someone who can help you.

Below is a collection of useful things to remember when you feel you need some psychic help and protection.

a. Ground yourself.
b. Centre yourself.
c. Close down your psychic centres.
d. Ask for help and guidance.   .
e. Do something active: sing, dance, go for a run.
f. Take a shower or a bath, and change into fresh clothes.
g. Send the energy away.
h. Do some protection exercises.

There are many creative ways of working with our energy systems, and each person has to find what works best for him. If we believe something will work, then that will greatly help it to work. Each individual can create his own exercises, that feel right to him, and allow him to refine his awareness in new ways.

Fig. 16.5

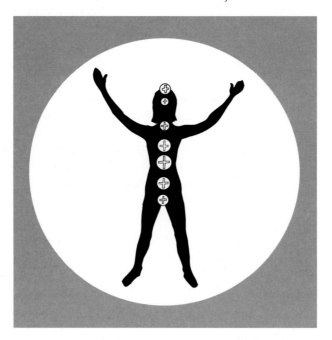

Protection using the Circle of Light

Chapter Seventeen

Coming Into Balance

The whole crux of economic life – and indeed of life in general – is that it constantly requires the living reconciliation of opposites which, in strict logic, are irreconcilable.

F. Schumacher

One effect of learning the Alexander technique is an improvement in posture, though Alexander teachers do not like to be described as teachers of improved posture. The word 'posture' suggests something rather static, a position robbed of movement and flow. An Alexander teacher is concerned with movement in the body, even when the body is still. The 'posture' of a person is usually seen as something quite superficial, an outer garment we wear to conceal an inner truth. As I mention in the introduction to this book, I spent a year or so of my youth 'trying' to achieve a posture badge, a good example of endgaining. The effect of this was to add an additional layer of misuse to my already poorly co-ordinated body. 'Posturing' suggests artificiality, something you put on to cover up the mess underneath. The Alexander technique works the other way round. By refining the sensitive mechanisms of balance it helps to change the mess underneath, so that the posture is a true reflection of inner balance. Alexander teachers prefer to describe the technique in terms of balance rather than posture. 'Balance' is a word that does not mislead in the way that 'posture' does, and it has implications which go far beyond the purely physical.

Our language is full of pairs of opposites. Think of an adjective or adverb and you will probably find its opposing word coming to mind quite easily. If we want to describe something that is balanced in the centre of a continuum, we often have to do it through the use of negatives, such as 'not too fast, not too slow'. Our vocabulary for the balanced median quality is often clumsy and cumbersome. Language is a reflection of our thoughts, and our thoughts are a reflection of our way of being, and 'being in balance' is a fairly new social idea, albeit a very popular one today, in the alternative health and growth movement.

Balanced Attention

The Alexander technique begins with a process of self-observation. For many people this involves turning their attention inwards more because they are habitually pre-occupied with their outwards attention. It is common for people to be totally caught up with events external to their inner state of being. Alternatively, when people study meditation techniques they may then become totally focused on internal events. With this technique we maintain a balance between the two states, which could be called a state of 'double attention', or of 'meditation in action'. This requires a balance between attention to what is going on inside the body and what is going on outside the body at the same time. In other words to be in a balanced state of awareness we need to learn to be aware of our internal states, but equally aware of our environment.

Thoughts and Feelings

Our awareness of what is happening both inside and outside us is sensory information, which can be experienced through the kinaesthetic sense, the internal and external sense organs, and our emotions. We can bring this information into our consciousness and balance it with our thoughts of what we want to create in our internal and external situations. We can then act from choice, rather than react from habit. Thoughts and feelings then work together in a state of creative flow.

Antagonistic Flow of the Muscles

Working with our thoughts we learn to balance the head on the spine, in such a way that we do not pull the head back and down. When we direct the head forwards and up, it allows the small sub-occipital muscles at the back of the head to lengthen and release, balanced by the weight of the forwards direction of the head. In this way we use the action of gravity through the head to create a lengthening down the spine. At the same time we balance the muscles in the front and the back of the neck, by directing the head to go up. If the head went forwards and down there would be contraction of the muscles down the front of the neck, and if it went backwards and down there would be contraction of the muscles down the back of the neck. And so with the power of thought we can create a mechanically advantageous relationship of balance, the muscles lengthening and releasing at the back and front of the neck, and potentially throughout the body as a whole.

We can go on to create this balance of the muscles throughout the body, using the Alexander directions, balancing the effect of gravity against some muscles, and balancing antagonistic pairs of muscles so that each set of muscles is as lengthened and released as possible, without creating contraction in the opposing muscles.

Gravity and Levity

Another perspective on balance in the body is to see the force of gravity in balance with the force of levity. Newton first defined the downward force of gravity, and he also postulated the scientific law that 'Action and Reaction are equal and opposite'. Applying this to our bodies means that as we stand with our feet placed on the earth, the weight of our bodies acting as a force downwards into the earth, we are supported by an equal and opposite force that is directed upwards through our feet into our bodies. This could be called the force of levity. If there were no such force we would simply sink down into the centre of the earth. So the pressure on our feet can be seen as the action and reaction of the force of gravity downwards, and the force of levity upwards. Balancing these two forces throughout the body would be another way of describing the work of the Alexander technique.

'Being' and 'Doing'

In order to bring about a creative antagonistic flow throughout the muscles in our body we use our minds in two ways. We inhibit habitual tendencies, and direct new desirable ones. In this way we are balancing two vital neurological functions, those of inhibition and excitation. Without inhibition a person is constantly reacting habitually to stimuli, suffering from over-stimulation of the nervous system. Without direction or volition, there is simply no motivation, nowhere to go, with a resulting tendency to muscular collapse. There are two parts to the body's autonomic nervous system, the sympathetic and the parasympathetic nervous systems. These operate antagonistically, in that the sympathetic nervous system stimulates the body, and the parasympathetic nervous system relaxes it. The sympathetic nervous system is able to increase the heart rate, raise blood-pressure, decrease the peristaltic action of the gut, all actions which are useful when the body is responding to stimulation, whereas the

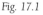
Fig. 17.1

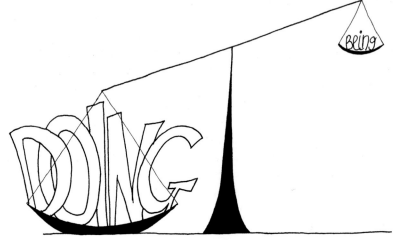

'The Unbearable Lightness of Being'

parasympathetic nervous system reverses those activities, by decreasing the heart rate, lowering the blood pressure, and increasing the peristaltic action of the gut so that digestion of food can take place. The sympathetic nervous system governs our 'doing' activity. It pumps adrenaline into the system, according to how much energy we need for any particular task, whereas the parasympathetic nervous system governs the involuntary 'being' activity of the body, the digestion of food, the conservation of energy. People under stress find the sympathetic nervous system is too dominant, and needs to be brought more into balance with the parasympathetic nervous system. One aspect of the Alexander Technique is balancing our 'being' and our 'doing' in this way.

Ends and Means

The ends we wish to gain must be balanced by the means whereby we gain them, another of the important principles of Alexander's method. Paying attention to the process we are going through involves being in the present moment, consciously inhibiting the unwanted habits of the past and any interfering fears or desires about the future, while directing positive desires about the future to come about. And so the balancing act becomes more subtle and complex.

Left and Right Hemispheres of the Brain

Many other balancing acts are going on when a person is operating with good use. Being aware of one's inner feeling state, as well as of the outside environment, is in itself a way of balancing the left and right hemispheres of the brain. The right hemisphere deals with the emotions and sensations while the left hemisphere can make logical observations about those feelings and about the outside world, as a result of which a person can operate from informed and reasoned choice, rather than from habit. Alexander called this 'constructive conscious control'. Bringing into left brain consciousness the rich and multifaceted information of the right brain is one of the most important balancing acts of our time.

Masculine and Feminine

Another polarity is frequently used to explain our behaviour. We all have a male and female principle operating within us, no matter what sex we are individually. The male principle is the outward, active, 'doing' energy, and the female principle is the inward, receptive, 'being' energy. The Chinese taoist philosophy contains the same concept, the male principle being called 'Yang' and the female principle 'Yin'. What I find interesting in this antagonism is that the visual symbols that we use for male and female suggest two of the ways in which we balance ourselves through the Alexander technique. The masculine symbol suggests 'Forwards and up', the primary direction for the head in relation to the spine, while the female principle suggests grounding, the downwards action of gravity.

Fig. 17.2

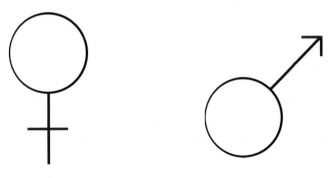

Female symbol   Male symbol

Balancing the Whole Person

To be in a state of balance does not always involve juggling with only two alternatives. From the above examples it is clear that many aspects of balance have to be considered at the same time. And the concept of balance applies to much more than the way we use our minds and bodies. It is really about the way we lead the whole of our lives, inwardly and outwardly. Our lives are full of interesting alternative possibilities. A person usually needs to give time and energy to her work, to her partner, to her family, to being with friends, to spending time on her own, to housework, to exercise, to rest, to leisure and creative pursuits, and with all these activities and more, there needs to be a balance between 'being' and 'doing', so that life is not just moving from one active role to another, which in itself is very stressful. Learning how to live a balanced life is very important to the art of changing.

I have found one of the best ways of understanding the psychological aspects of balance is to work with the mundane level of the chakras. The Alexander technique helps to integrate and balance the flow of energy through the chakras, and if in addition we become conscious of the different parts of ourselves that each chakra controls, we can help the balancing process by being more consciously aware of our needs. For example, if a person tends to judge himself very harshly, this is due to an imbalance in the third chakra. By acknowledging his own power and value, the emotive negative judgements of the third chakra can be transformed into the wisdom of the sixth chakra, so that a harsh judgmental attitude can transform into a keen sense of discrimination. If in addition he is developing the acceptance and trust of the heart chakra energy, the critical appraisal of the sixth chakra will be balanced by love and acceptance, and so the attitude of the person will contain a balance of loving acceptance and discrimination. The 'harsh judge' then becomes the 'helpful guide', a much easier sub-personality to live with. We all tend to have a sceptic within us who needs to be reconciled with a faithful devotee. To the sceptic anything can be discounted. To the faithful anything can be accepted. As we balance our energy, our analytical scrutiny is balanced by a faith and openness to new ideas. This is similar to reconciling the critic and the creator within us, so that our own new ideas are treated with trust and openness, and also with discrimination and critical awareness.

Refining one's self-observation is essential to all growth work. Without it, change is likely to be forced and superficial. With it, one may stop wanting to change, or may want to change in very different ways. People often know who they want to be, but they don't know who they are. For example, there are many people who would like to be great mountain climbers. They may wish to do this to prove to themselves that they can survive (Root chakra), or because climbing mountains gives them deep satisfaction (Sacral chakra), or because it will give them social status and add to their achievements (Solar Plexus chakra), or they may find climbing mountains gives them a great sense of love and oneness with the world around them (Heart chakra), or they may want to communicate the experience to others (Throat chakra), or they may be fascinated by the geology of mountains, and wish to study it fully (Eye chakra) or they may experience God and their own divinity, in an egoless way, through this experience (Crown chakra).

Most likely there will be a combination of many of these reasons in the motivation of a great mountain climber. Every activity we are involved in stimulates some of the chakras. But unless we know ourselves, by knowing which chakras are functioning well, and which are overactive or underactive, we cannot tell whether a particular activity is bringing us into balance, or stimulating an already overactive part of ourselves. If we have an overactive third chakra and we constantly take on more challenges to stimulate it more, then this will not be so good for our energy system as it would be if we turned our energy to an underactive chakra, possibly the sacral chakra, and found ways in which we could be more centred and nourished through that centre.

By developing our conscious awareness we can discover whether we are reinforcing habitual behaviour or not. As we learn to balance our chakras, so that none is neglected and none extremely overactive, then the desire to change will become simply a desire to be oneself, and to develop one's potential. Change can be seen as the removal of interferences to an improved use of the self, rather than a new suit of clothes which is put on over the same old self.

The balancing of logically irreconcilable opposites within our psyches is a rich and complex process. Often before balance is achieved the pendulum swings unsteadily from one extreme to the other, until it oscillates gently around the centre point of its path. As I discussed in the chapter on emotions, integrating a hitherto repressed or neglected aspect of oneself may mean that for a time the new element is very dominant and obsessive.

We cannot short cut this process. Many people are so uncomfortable about the blocks and interferences in the lower chakras that they prefer to cut the energy off from that part of themselves. This is understandable, especially for those people who are aware that they are radiating out their own energy field, and they don't want to fill the world with their 'difficult' energy. But if we cut off the energy flow from our lower chakras, we cut off our instincts and our feelings, and we radiate out that repressive energy we are creating within ourselves. Energy does not know how to lie. We cannot pretend to be perfect. If we do, then we simply radiate pretence. If we cut off the creative flow between our thoughts and our feelings we cut off our inspiration. As some-one once said, 'If you want to light a bright fire, you've got to dig the coal'.

The whole of human life fluctuates between different antagonisms, the inspiration and expiration of our breathing, the contraction and expansion of our muscles, the forces of gravity and levity, the processes of birth and death, and many more. If we can learn to experience the flow between these physiological antagonisms as creative and constructive, then we can balance the inner conflicts within our psyches with a simi-lar rationale.

THE ART OF CHANGING

You can never step in the same river twice. Heraclitus

Why do most people want to change, and often, at the same time, want to resist change? What do we mean by change? The world we live in changes all the time. Living itself is a process of changing. We can never step in the same river twice because, not only has the river changed, but we also have changed. Nothing remains the same from moment to moment. As Heraclitus also put it, everything is in a state of continuous flux.

All living beings are in a continuous process of growth or decay death and rebirth. Not only does the individual change, but the world around her changes too. When I was in San Francisco, I remember watching a play performed by three women about the problem of being fat. One woman clutched a jar of peanut butter and addressed it longingly: 'Everything in my life has changed except you. No wonder I rush to you for comfort whenever something new happens.' Many people find it painful and dis-turbing to adapt to change. As one person cynically remarked, 'Life's difficult, and then you die'. Fixed habitual responses don't allow us to flow with the changes that occur in and around us.

A kaleidoscope is an example of an object that adapts perfectly to change. With each alteration in position, with each change in the gravitational field on the pieces inside the tube, the pieces move, and the pattern changes to a beautiful new arrangement. This is an example of passive change. The kaleidoscope responds passively to the action of the world upon it. But human beings are not kaleidoscopes and although we do have to learn to respond flexibly to the changes that take place around us, when we talk about change this is not primarily what we mean. We also have an active prin-ciple of change, as does any living being. Just as oak trees from tiny acorns grow, so the human body moves through its life from the foetus, through many stages of growth, development and decay until it becomes a corpse. Life is a transforming process. An active principle of change is at work within us, in addition to the changes going on around us in the outside world, to which we have to make continual adjustments. And this active principle is expressed through the physical, emotional, mental and spiritual aspects of our being.

Balancing the Principle of Balance

The principle of a dynamic internal balance is central to all life forms, and the tendency to maintain this balanced state is called the principle of homeostasis. Every living organism fluctuates between different sets of variables, adapting to changes in environment by alterations within those variables. We have a range of possibilities in such variables as our heart rate, our temperature and our breathing, all of which move to an extreme when it is necessary to adapt to some new condition, and then tend to return to their resting rates as soon as possible. If we exceed the extremes of any variable, then we are likely to die. And yet it is equally natural for us to push our physiological limits, as Olympic sportsmen and women do every day. Fairly recent biological research suggests that the principle of homeostasis is balanced by another principle, that of the desire for the organism to transform to a higher state of being, which in effect is an interpretation of the process of evolution. So our tendency to bring ourselves into balance is in itself balanced by our tendency to move towards a more complex organization of the life form. Although this is a theory about biological species, by analogy it can be applied to the self-development of each individual human being: inwardly we are drawn towards growth and self-transformation and at the same time we need to be grounded, integrated and in balance.

This creative antagonism is reflected in the structure of the human body. Because the weight of the head is forwards of the point of pivot where the head balances on the spine (See *Fig. 6.1*, page 83), we have to constantly maintain a state of dynamic equilibrium of the head upon the spine in order to remain in balance. In other words a balanced state, such as standing, is not static but a constant interplay between rest and change.

Human walking is a unique activity during which the body, step by step, teeters on the edge of catastrophe.

Napier, *The antiquity of human walking*

In order to make simple movements such as in walking, we throw the body out of gravitational balance and then save it from falling, creating an even greater dynamic interplay between the principles of rest and change. This interplay is also reflected in the relationship between inhibition and direction. Inhibition is a pause which allows us to return to the point of balance and rest, while direction moves us forwards to a new changed state of being.

Every living organism is subject to these two antagonistic principles of homeostasis and self-transformation. Although the formulation of these two balancing principles is a biological hypothesis, as a philosophical concept it is as old as the hills. Aristotle, when defining the nature of living beings wrote, 'Each of them has within itself a principle of change and rest.' It is natural for a living being to seek balance and integration, and at the same time to seek self-transformation, to move to a higher level of consciousness. This is the experience of being alive, the activity of the life force.

Balance and Growth Through the Chakras

In the womb and in the first months of life we maintain homeostasis through the survival mechanisms of the root chakra. From this base we transform ourselves through the second chakra by reaching out for pleasurable contact and nourishment, once again integrating this transformation, centering ourselves in the sacral chakra. So then we are integrating our instincts, our connection to the earth, our past and, through the second chakra, our sensations and emotions, our present feeling situation.

As we move upwards through the chakras there continues an experience of growth and self-transformation. At each stage of growth, the transformation has to be integrated and the whole energy system brought to a new higher level of balance and homeostasis. In an ideal situation the growth proceeds as follows:

The third chakra is one of personal growth, measured in terms of achievements, successes and failures. We then progress to the fourth chakra where we move to a transpersonal level, experiencing our individuality as part of a larger pattern, where self-acceptance can be felt as a logical necessity, because what is, is, and everything is worthwhile and valid. From this position of acceptance the development to the fifth chakra is one of true communication. One hears truly, without the distortions of imbalanced lower chakras, and one speaks truly, expressing the unique and undistorted reality of the self. Moving through to the sixth chakra we transform our vision and understanding of reality, we see clearly, our seeing is not distorted by our personal energy imbalances, our needs and hopes and fears, until finally, through development of the crown chakra, we understand the whole.

In the heart chakra we experience 'the whole' at a feeling level, and in the crown chakra we know it and we become it. We are no longer governed by the physical, emotional and mental bad habits of the past, but have discovered our own autonomy, our own Godliness. This is total, constructive, conscious control and freedom. We radiate out our pure and unique life force, and are open to the creative flow around us, which we are part of. We respond flexibly, with openness, integrating this flow with the clarity of our own inner flow, direction, and centredness, and experiencing the interaction as inspiration. We can respond to that inspiration by moving forwards into the future, without losing our awareness of the present and our contact with the earth. Our actions are balanced, and we are transforming ourselves at the same time. We are not living in a fantasy world, nor are we stuck in a rut. We are poised between heaven and earth, moving forwards in the direction of our 'positive' ideals, while accepting and integrating the 'negative' aspects of ourselves. The energies flowing through us represent the forces of levity and gravity, of inspiration and expiration, of expansion and contraction and many other creative antagonisms. And from the subtle balancing of these energies we are able to transform ourselves; and as we transform ourselves we transform the world around us.

This process of growth and development is a natural part of being alive. Unfortunately the process is not as ideal as the way in which I have outlined it here. Distortions and interferences in one chakra will affect the flow through the chakras around it, but it is possible to let go of interferences and distortions by learning how to change in a constructive way.

THE NEW AGE

May you live in interesting times. Ancient Chinese Curse

There is a lot of talk about how, with the arrival of a new millennium, we are entering a New Age. There is also a lot of talk about how unlikely we are to survive through the new millennium because of the many ways in which we are destroying the earth upon which we live. In the words of a Greenpeace pamphlet:

Planet Earth is 4,600 million years old. If we condense this inconceivable time-span into an understandable concept, we can liken Earth to a person of 46 years of age.

Nothing is known about the first 7 years of this person's life, and whilst only scattered information exists about the middle span we know that only at the age of 42 did the earth begin to flower.

Dinosaurs and the great reptiles did not appear until one year ago, when the planet was 45. Mammals arrived only 8 months ago; in the middle of last week man-like apes evolved into ape-like men, and at the weekend the last ice age enveloped the Earth. Modern man has been around for 4 hours. During the last hour Man discovered agriculture. The industrial revolution began a minute ago.

During those sixty seconds of biological time, modern man has made a rubbish tip of Paradise.

He has multiplied his numbers to plague proportions, caused the extinction of 500 species of animals, ransacked the planet for fuels and now stands like a brutish infant, gloating over this meteoric rise to ascendancy, on the brink of a war to end all wars and in danger of effectively destroying this oasis of life in the solar system.

On the other hand there is a very optimistic voice suggesting that the New Age will be an age of love and healing for ourselves and the planet; For example:

Your mission on earth at this time is to become who you really are. As you remember who you are you will awaken within others the remembrance of who they are. This effect will grow and grow and spread as a Fire of Realization across the once confused face of the Earth. At a specific Moment, soon to be reached, humanity and the Earth will lift into a higher level of existence and John the Beloved's Vision of A New Heaven and A New Earth will become fulfilled.

So be it. This is your mission. Now is the Time. 'Be Who You Are.

Acorn Publications

We are certainly living in interesting times. The changes moving through our world are affecting everything, from our economies, our institutions, social and family life, to the way we think about ourselves and the world itself.

Two scientific models are in use today as an explanation of man and the world. The older model is that of man as a machine. This idea originated in the 17th century in the scientific work of Descartes and Newton. Today this model is usually based upon the idea that man is like a complex computer, although the original machine that inspired Descartes' thinking was the clock. He saw the universe as an intricate piece of clockwork, which could be made to run smoothly by a God that existed separately from the machine. Similarly, man was like a clock that would run smoothly until it broke down and needed repairing, or throwing away. The effect of this model upon our methods of economy, education, healthcare, social welfare and our relationship to the rest of the planet has been profound. The original value of a scientific approach was gradually undermined by the soulless mechanistic perspective, to the extent that the 'God outside the machine', in which both Descartes and Newton sincerely believed, became logically dispensable. Today we are faced with many problems in all areas of our lives as a result of this kind of perspective.

The new model being used to explain the world is the model of a living organism. This is a fundamentally different approach to understanding ourselves and the universe. A living organism has its own active principle of change within it, its own ways of maintaining stability, through death and renewal of living cells. It does not require a mechanic to repair a breakdown. If the earth is a living organism, then we can be seen as cells within it, parts of a whole. This is similar to the model of the Universe as an energy system which I have been using. It emphasizes interaction and interrelationship. The boundaries between subjective and objective become less clear. God is no longer external to the operation, but immanent within it. God is the totality of creation, the life force, or the creative dancing energy throughout the universe, as in the vision of Eastern Mysticism and the New Physics.

Such enormous changes in mental perspective inevitably create great changes at a physical level, and as these new ideas and directions enter our collective thinking, the New Age is clearly underway. Looking at the model of the world as a living organism, it is quite easy to imagine that, in addition to human beings operating as individual cells within the organism, humanity itself is also a living organism, moving through her evolutionary process. Once again the chakras can be helpful in understanding this. In the beginning of human life on earth, the energy required was one of survival, the root chakra of the human race was activated. We lived by our instincts and our survival mechanisms. As we mastered the skills of survival, particularly from the beginning of agricultural development, there was time for more pleasure and nourishment in our lives. Tribal culture developed and the sense of belonging to a tribe which would protect and support you. So the second chakra of the human race began to be energized. The third chakra began to open with the coming of the industrial revolution, the discovery of how powerful and successful we can be, what great achievements we have made. And now, with the New Age, the human race has the opportunity to open the heart centre, to understand that we are all connected and interrelated, that we can use our power responsibly, to take care of the planet, to love and accept all of life, and to heal ourselves and the world around us.

One of the first things that inevitably happens when a person becomes powerful is that he misuses his power. When he has misused it he is then in a position to learn how to be responsible with it. It would certainly appear that the living organism of the human race is misusing its power. I would like to think that we now have the opportunity of learning how to be responsible with our power; and it is this change in our consciousness which heralds in the New Age.

The Growth Movement

The development of the Human Potential or 'Growth' movement, in which I include the Alternative Health movement coincides with this changing process which is part of our planetary development. The interest in new healing techniques that emphasize the 'whole' person, and in techniques for developing individual potential, self-development and personal growth, have snowballed dramatically in the last fifty years. Alexander was ahead of his time, being one of the first people to write about new concepts such as the unity of mind and body and the need for balance at many levels, ideas which are now the common currency of the growth movement. One central theme of his work was the concept of how we use ourselves, and how we use ourselves and the planet is now a central theme in the New Age movement. The Alexander technique is very much a part of the Growth movement, an important living cell within the larger living organism of the growth network. Like all living cells it needs to maintain its individuality, while accepting its interrelationship and connection to other types of growth and healing work.

The energies of the heart chakra are essential to the New Age, which is why there is such an emphasis on wholeness, healing and balance, all heart qualities. All the alternative health and growth techniques and therapies place an emphasis on the wholeness of the human being, although it is interesting to notice the different areas in which different techniques direct their attention.

Many healing techniques, such as Acupuncture and Homeopathy, see their work as balancing the energies in the human body, and parallels can be drawn between these disciplines and the Alexander Technique. The ancient Chinese philosophy upon which acupuncture is based recognises Ch'i energy, which is differentiated into two antagonistic forces of Yin and Yang, Yin being the principle of rest, of integration, of conservation of energy, and Yang being the principle of growth, expansion, and outwardly directed energy. Subtle balancing of the Yin and Yang energy flows through the body brings about an improvement in the overall Ch'i. Homeopathy finds remedies with a vibration which resonates with the vibration of the patient and this resonance encourages a healing process which energizes the 'vital force' of the patient. Many healers who work with their hands describe their work as 'energy balancing'. In many ways the alternative health movement works to assist the individual to rediscover an internal balance which then allows her to grow, develop her potential and enjoy life more fully, and the Alexander Technique contributes to this exciting work.

Psychotherapies of various types, and counselling techniques, work more directly with the emotions than do the more physically oriented healing techniques. It is interesting that the Alexander Technique, while not traditionally working at the emotional level, nevertheless shares something with these methods, in that it sets out to teach, rather than to heal. 'Emotional therapists', as I shall call them for simplicity, are interested in helping their clients develop skills that can be applied to everyday life. They help to develop the ability to be self-aware and take responsibility for oneself, giving more attention to emotional and mental habits, where the Alexander Teacher tends to emphasize physical and mental habits.

Fig. 17.3

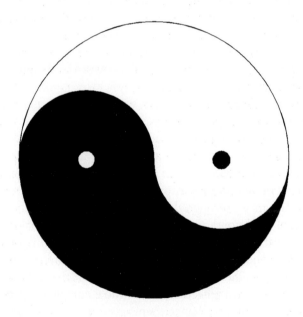

Yin Yang Symbol

Some growth techniques focus directly on energizing the chakras. A lot of breathing techniques do this. While energizing the chakras may be valuable, it depends whether particular chakras are overactive or underactive. It is important to remember that stimulation needs to be balanced by integration, and to check that this is occurring with the particular therapy or therapist. It is also important to remember that breathing is a natural automatic function and interfering with the breathing may develop harmful habits.

With all the workshops available today it helps to assess them in terms of what chakras they are emphasizing. Courses that focus on relationships emphasize the second chakra. Assertiveness training courses emphasize the third chakra. Both these types of course also require the energy of the fifth chakra to be developed in order to improve communication. Workshops which use a lot of visualization are emphasizing the fifth and sixth chakras, sometimes in relation to the lower chakras. And some courses focus primarily on the heart chakra. Meditation courses usually have a spiritual bias, although meditation is a very direct method of allowing the energy to flow through the chakras by means of positive attention.

There are many facets to the health and growth movement, and it is useful to assess the different approaches by reference to the chakras. Then, if you have some idea through your own visualizations and observations which of your chakras are underactive and which overactive, you can decide which courses or therapies are going to be of most help to you personally.

The growth movement is an energy system within the greater energy system of the human race. It is not perfect, being a reflection of its time, but it is an exciting historical development offering inspiration and assistance to individuals who are searching for healing and growth. As it grows, and as more and more individuals become more self-aware and more able to balance and integrate their energies, then the influence of this movement will spread, through word of mouth, the media, and books like this one, but also simply through the energy transformations that are taking place in the living being of the human race. As we learn to heal and balance ourselves, we will know how to heal and balance our environment, as each is part of the other. I am not suggesting that nothing should be done now, that we must wait until we are all perfectly balanced. On the contrary, I am saying that the actions of environmentalists and other activists are a reflection of the whole energy structure, as too are the actions of individuals seeking to change themselves. Each individual will follow, in a more or less distorted way, the direction of his own life force which will move him to realize himself, to become more real, and to do what his inspiration suggests is right for him to do.

Your Body Your Temple

The song that I came to sing remains unsung to this day.
I have spent my days in stringing and unstringing my instrument.
The time has not come true, the words have not been rightly set; only there is the
agony of wishing in my heart.
The blossom has not opened; only the mind is sighing by.

Rabindranath Tagore

Pete came to see me because he suffered from constant back pain. He was in his mid-twenties. Four years earlier he had been registered disabled and unfit to work, because of the pain. He spent over three quarters of his day lying down, because as soon as he got up to do the necessary tasks such as eating and washing he was in extreme pain. It was difficult for him to come to see me, but fortunately there was a quite rapid improvement in his condition in the first few weeks of lessons.

Pete had spent most of those four years lying on his tummy with his arms and head over the end of the bed writing a book about the history of the local railway line, which is now published.* He could not stay in this position for long, because after a while it became painful, so then he would move slowly onto his back and do the reading and research for the book. He didn't lack persistence.

After a few weeks of lessons he was able to get about much better, and to remain with his spine in the vertical without the pain getting too bad, but there was a resistance and rigidity in his body which was blocking further progress. We began to talk about his plans if he became well enough to work again. At first he seemed relieved at the thought of doing any job at all, after so much forced immobility. Previously, he had worked in an office, but had not enjoyed it. I suggested that sometimes we get pain in order to teach us something, and that if we persist in doing things that we don't really like then that can cause the pain. We looked at what was working well for him in his life, and what was difficult.

One of Pete's difficulties was that he lived on one of the busiest roads leading into the town, and he could not stand the sound of the traffic. He said he would like to live in the middle of a forest somewhere, out of earshot of all traffic; that he would love to work for the Forestry Commission or some similar organization because he had a passion for the countryside and would like to help take care of it in some way.

Today he owns a little piece of forested wilderness in the middle of Wales, where he

---

*The Birmingham and Gloucestershire Railway, P. J. Long & Rev. W. Awdry, published by Alan Sutton.

has parked his caravan. He has set up in self-employment as a landscaper for practical conservation, and although it is hard physical work his back gives him less trouble than it did when he lived on a noisy street. He still gets problems from time to time, usually when he is mentally and emotionally stressed, rather than due to the physical stress of his work, and particularly when he has to listen to noisy machinery.

What Pete says about all this is that his back got better when he 'sorted out the spiritual problems'. He realized at some point that the pain in his body was trying to tell him something, and when he listened and took seriously the underlying yearnings of his soul for a different sort of life, something deep inside himself released, and the pain and rigidity went away. Now his life not only satisfies him personally, he also feels he is making a contribution to the planet through his work.

It is not very often in a person's life that he will take time to really consider why he is alive and what are the meaning and purpose behind his existence. Often such a search for meaning only occurs when a person goes through some kind of personal crisis, such as a painful or debilitating dis-ease in the body, or emotional trauma of some sort. It was a crisis in my health that gave me the opportunity to stop working in the theatre and begin training as an Alexander teacher, and for Alexander himself it was a serious voice problem that put him on the path to his great discoveries. An imbalance in the energy system can lead to a search for a higher level of balance, integration and growth.

Sometimes when a student starts experiencing the changes brought about by the Alexander Technique the door is opened to these kinds of spiritual questions. Working with the technique, a student begins to develop his self-awareness, to stop endgaining, to clear away some of the energy blockages from the past and to live life more in the present. This experience often leads naturally to a questioning about the values of life, and a searching for new values, for what has inner value, for what will make life truly fulfiling and meaningful. These are the questions that are being asked in all the spiritual disciplines of our age.

The original meaning of spirit is 'breath'. We inspire and expire the breath of life into our bodies from the moment they are born to the moment they die. The spirit also means the life-force of a person, and this life-force is something much greater than our material bodies. Like the breath it flows through us, connecting us to the greater whole, to the energy system of the universe. And the energy of the whole remains constant. It transforms, it dances, but it does not die. Each particular person's energy system receives inspiration from the larger whole of which it is a part. An awareness of the Spiritual dimension of life is an awareness of this greater whole, which 'inspires' us. When we start 'sorting out the spiritual problems', we begin listening to this inspiration. We stop resisting or interfering with that creative flow of energy which helps us move through our lives in the direction in which it is right for us to go.

Each individual has the possibility of taking care of his own system, bringing it into balance, and allowing the energy flowing through to inspire him to work in whatever way is uniquely appropriate to his system; in other words allowing him to be truly himself. The way we balance the energy of our system will be different for each of us. Each individual is unique, offering his special contribution as an energy system to the whole energy system of the universe. Each one of us has a part to play, and the more self-aware we become the clearer we can be about what our part is in the great cosmic drama. The less we suffer from faulty sensory and emotional appreciation, the more we can trust the inspiration about what is 'right' for us.

The Alexander Technique offers a great contribution to this changing world, because it offers a methodology of how to change. By developing our awareness of how we are and of how we are using ourselves our level of consciousness is raised. Having increased that awareness we are in a position to stop reacting habitually, whether it be from physical habits of misuse, or emotional and mental habits based on unconscious drives. We can experience our sensory and emotional responses fully, make them conscious, so that our actions then can be based on choice, taking into account all the information available to us. We inhibit reaction and direct action. This is the only way genuine change can occur. Unwanted habitual reactions interfere with a balanced flow of energy. As Alexander said, if we remove these interferences 'the right thing will do itself'. We then have the opportunity to balance our whole selves, allowing the creative flow of the life-force to inspire us.

These principles, applied to our physical use can make the body a temple worthy of the soul. Applied to our energy system as a whole they offer a means whereby we can take part in our own evolution.

'Look', said Siddhartha softly to Govinda, 'there is the Buddha'.

Govinda looked at the monk in the yellow cowl, who could not be distinguished in any way from the hundreds of other monks, and yet Govinda soon recognised him . . . He wore his gown and walked along exactly like the other monks, but his face and his step, his peaceful downward glance, his peaceful downward hanging hand, and every finger of his hand spoke of peace, spoke of completeness, sought nothing, imitated nothing.

Siddhartha looked attentively at the Buddha's head, at his shoulders, at his feet, at his still downward-hanging hand, and it seemed to him that in every joint of every finger of his hand there was knowledge; they spoke, breathed, radiated truth.

Hermann Hesse. *Siddhartha,*

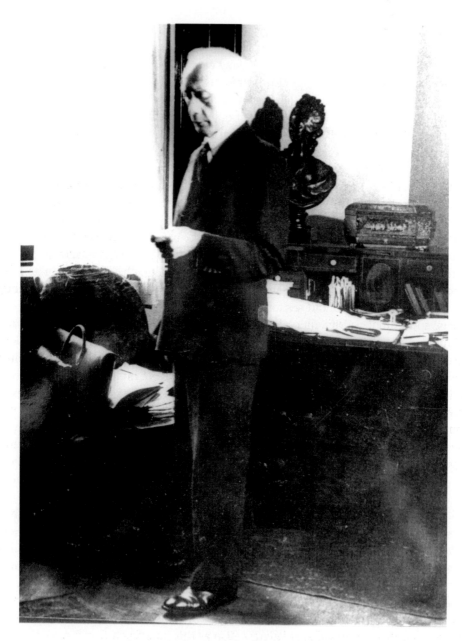

Frederick Matthias Alexander (1869–1955)

APPENDIX

A Short Biography of Frederick Matthias Alexander

Frederick Matthias Alexander was an Australian. He was born in 1869 and grew up in the small town of Wynyard on the North Western coast of Tasmania. He was the eldest of eight children.

Several significant themes stand out in Alexander's childhood. Alexander had a deep and enduring relationship with his mother who was a very strong character. She acted as the local nurse and midwife, saddling up her horse and racing off to help when the local doctors needed her. She was self-taught and from her he learned self-sufficiency and the determination to find his own solutions to the problems of his life.

He was an extremely difficult child to 'school', partly because he didn't respond well to formal education and was an awkward pupil, and partly because he suffered from respiratory problems in his early years. The teacher of the local school offered to tutor Alexander in the evenings and this was the only education he received. Possibly this was a blessing in disguise because his individualistic nature and enquiring mind were not thwarted by traditional teaching methods. Alexander was an intelligent child and won prizes for the school, despite his lack of attendance.

Because he did not attend school, he was able to indulge his love of the country and in particular his passion for horses. He spent a lot of time with horses, and developed the skills of careful observation of their movements and of the handling of these sensitive creatures, skills which were to be helpful to him later.

His other passion was for the theatre, and particularly for Shakespeare. When Alexander was seventeen he began his first job in the office of a Tin Mining Company in Mount Bischoff. He was sorry to leave his country life behind. He occupied his spare time with amateur dramatics and teaching himself to play the violin. After three years he had saved enough money to go to Melbourne, where he stayed with an uncle. Of this time he says, 'For three months or so, I was chiefly interested in seeing and hearing all that was best in the theatre, the art galleries and in music. By this time I had decided to train myself as a Reciter.' Also at this time Sarah Bernhardt was touring Australia and he went to see her twice a day.

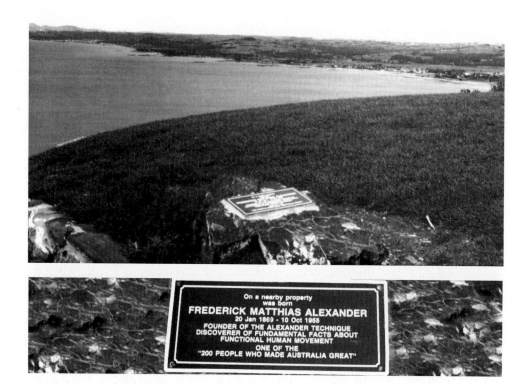

On a nearby property
was born
FREDERICK MATTHIAS ALEXANDER
20 Jan 1869 - 10 Oct 1955
FOUNDER OF THE ALEXANDER TECHNIQUE
DISCOVERER OF FUNDAMENTAL FACTS ABOUT
FUNCTIONAL HUMAN MOVEMENT
ONE OF THE
"200 PEOPLE WHO MADE AUSTRALIA GREAT"

Memorial commemorating Alexander's birthplace

Alexander embarked upon his career as a recitationist with some success. Like many actors today he sought out engagements, and when times were hard, he took odd jobs here and there to earn some extra cash. In time he gained recognition and he formed his own theatre company. But his career as an actor was marred by a tendency he had developed to become hoarse and lose his voice during a performance.

It was this difficulty that was the turning point and, from another point of view, the great opportunity in Alexander's life. He tried every way he could to solve his voice problem. His doctor advised him to rest his voice before a performance, and on one occasion he rested his voice for two whole weeks before going on stage, only to discover that he still became hoarse during his recitation. His doctor could offer no further advice although he agreed that it must be something that he was doing when he was reciting. Alexander decided to find out what he was doing on stage that was causing him the problem.

At this point Alexander embarked upon a process of self-observation that went on for about nine or ten years. He worked with mirrors, developing in more and more depth and detail an understanding of the use of the self. He discovered what he was doing that caused his vocal problems, and how to develop improved coordination throughout the body, by means of his method or technique.

During this time he continued to live the life of an actor, but increasingly other actors would come to him for help with their voice and breathing problems, and Alexander's career began to move from acting to teaching others his unique technique. He taught in Melbourne and then in Sydney, where for four years he was the director of the Sydney Dramatic and Operatic Conservatorium, and then in 1904 he travelled to London to make his technique known there.

In London, actors flocked to Alexander for lessons and he became known as 'the protector of the London theatre'. His pupils included famous performers such as Sir Henry Irving and Viola Tree. Sometimes he would work with the stars in their dressing rooms before the start of the show. There were many famous and respected people who became devotees of the Alexander technique, including George Bernard Shaw, Aldous Huxley, Sir Stafford Cripps, and later in America, John Dewey, and many more.

During the first world war Alexander went to New York to teach, and so spread the knowledge of his method further abroad. After the war he returned to England, but moved backwards and forwards between England and America for the next few years. His brother Albert Redden Alexander had learned to teach the technique and worked alongside him until 1924 when 'AR' stayed in America and Frederick Matthias, or 'FM', as he was called, settled back in England, where he established a school for children from the ages of three to eight, based on the Alexander principles.

He began the first training school for teachers of the Alexander technique in 1930. Being a self-taught man he was not skilled at teaching others to teach what he had learnt through self-observation and experiment, but slowly new teachers of the Alexander technique became qualified and the teaching of the Alexander technique became more widespread. The second world war disrupted his work in England and so once again he transferred his entire practice, including the school for children, to America, returning to England in 1943. Four years later at the age of seventy-nine he suffered from a stroke which paralysed the left side of his body but through using his technique he regained conscious control of this within a year, and returned to his teaching. He continued to teach until his death in 1955 at the age of eighty-six.

This brief outline covers the essential details of Alexander's career. I have omitted a great deal, such as his unhappy marriage to an Australian actress and his long and drawn out, although eventually successful, libel action against the South African government.

He never lost his passion for horses and horse-racing. Equally he never lost his love of the theatre, and at one point he thought the best way he could train teachers of the technique was to teach them how to perform Shakespeare, and he presented 'Hamlet' at the Old Vic and 'The Merchant of Venice' at Sadler's Wells. Unfortunately most of his student teachers had little talent and no desire to act and from the reviews of these plays this was apparent. As an actress myself, I think it is a pity that Alexander never produced a play with professional actors, during the latter part of his career, as I believe this would have resulted in an exciting evolution of acting technique. But if his work had developed in this direction there might never have been a generation of new teachers to pass on his discoveries, discoveries which are important for the well-being of the human race as a whole.

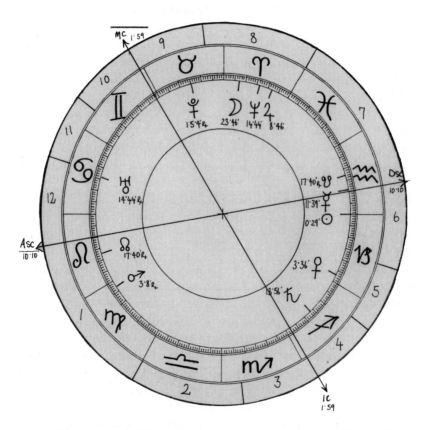

Natal horoscope of F. M. Alexander, using data given to one of his pupils

ADDRESSES

Audio Cassette Tape
As described on page 10, there is an audio cassette tape which accompanies this book. The cassette is available through bookshops (ISBN 1 85398 131 1) or direct from Ashgrove Publishing, 3 Town Barton, Norton St Philip, Bath BA3 6LN, U.K. Telephone/Fax: 01373 834900

If you wish to work with an Alexander Technique teacher in your area contact one of the following Professional Associations of Alexander Teachers:

Society of Teachers of the Alexander Technique

STAT head office: (world-wide membership)
20 London House,
266 Fulham Road,
London SW10 9EL
Tel: 020 7351 0828
Fax: 020 7352 1556
email: enquiries@stat.org.uk
website: www.stat.org.uk

Australian Soc. of Teachers of the A.T.
(AUSTAT)
PO Box 716,
Darlinghurst,
NSW 2010, Australia
Tel: 61 3 8339 571
Fax: 61 3 9529 2372
email: ruthshoe@bigpond.com

Alexander Technique International
ATI offices:

UK: 66C Thurlestone Rd,
West Norwood,
London SE27 0PD
Tel. 070 7188 0253
email uk@ati-net.com

USA: (main headquarters)
1692 Massachusetts Avenue,
Cambridge, MA 02138,
USA
email usa@ati-net.com

Ireland: ireland@ati-net.ie
Norway: norway@ati-net.com
Sweden: sweden@ati-net.com

France: Tel: (+33) 01.43.35.10.48
Germany: germany@ati-net.com
Switzerland: switzerland@ati-net.com

Glen Park and Delia Hardy run 'Art of Changing' courses. For more information visit our website at http://www.glenpark.org.uk Or write: c/o Ashgrove Publishing

INDEX

CREDITS

Photographs:

David Broomby, pages 120, 121
Walter Carrington, page 118
Daniel J. Cox/naturalexposures.com, page 93
Gerry Cranham, pages 86, 87
Mel France, page 95
Richard and Sally Greenhill, pages 56, 144, 145
Delia Hardy, pages 127, 194, 195
John Kennaby, pages 52, 62, 84, 119, 142, 143, 157, 186, 201, 280
Hilary Thacker, pages 32, 123
The Mansell Collection, page 189
National Galleries of Scotland, page 139
The Oriental Museum, Durham, pages 199, 209
S.T.A.T., page 278

Additional illustrations:

David Lupton, page 176
Quest Books, 221, 222, 223, 224, 225
Rachel Stevens/ Robert Chandler, page 282

Published in Great Britain by
ASHGROVE PUBLICATIONS
an imprint of
HOLLYDATA PUBLISHERS LTD
55 Richmond Avenue
London N1 0LX

First published 1989
Reprinted 1989 Reprinted 1990
New edition 1991
Reprinted 1992, 1993, 1995, 1997, 1998
New Edition 2000

British Library Cataloguing in Publication Data

Park, Glen
The art of changing.
1 Physical fitness. Posture. Theories of Alexander, F. Matthias
I. Title
613.7'8'0924

ISBN 1-85398-130-3

Book Design by Brad Thompson
Cover Design by John Kennaby
Printed and bound in Malta by Interprint